TURNING
WEEDS *into*
WILD
FLOWERS

TURNING WEEDS *into* WILD FLOWERS

A True Story *of* FAITH, HOPE, *and* HEALING in the Face *of* Childhood Cancer

EMILY GOULD
ALEXIS GOULD STAFFORD

CFI

An imprint of Cedar Fort, Inc.

Springville, Utah

Photo on page 246 taken by Jennifer Staniforth
Photo on page 247 taken by Gracee Paige Horrocks

ISBN 13: 978-1-4621-2269-1

Published by CFI, an imprint of Cedar Fort, Inc.
2373 W. 700 S., Springville, UT 84663
Distributed by Cedar Fort, Inc., www.cedarfort.com

LIBRARY OF CONGRESS CATALOGING-IN-PUBLICATION DATA ON FILE

Cover design by Wes Wheeler
Cover design © 2018 Cedar Fort, Inc.
Edited and typeset by Jessilyn Peaslee and Nicole Terry

Printed in the United States of America

10 9 8 7 6 5 4 3 2 1

Printed on acid-free paper

To my mom, who planted the seed of faith in my heart
and watered it every chance she could; my sisters and
brothers, who grew alongside me; my grandparents, who still
remember my favorite flower; my beautiful children, Lex,
Cam, Liv, and Leah, who continually bring sunshine into
my world; and mostly to the love of my eternity, Kris, who
forever holds my hand and works so hard to make sure that
all of life's weeds turn into wildflowers.

—E. G.

To Katie with Love—
May you find peace in your soul,
Love in your heart,
and joy in all of life's journeys.
May all your weeds forever
become wildflowers.
— Emily Gould

Contents

Contents

Prologue

$\mathcal{B}$elieve it or not, this is a happy story. Not your typical sun-shine-and-endless-puppies kind of happy, but a story about true happiness. This story is about the kind of happiness that lasts—the kind that is founded on our responses to life, not our circum-stances. This type of happiness is not based on everything in life that is going right; rather, it is based on our choice to be happy when everything goes wrong. It is a happiness that is actively sought after, one that is earned.

Despite the happiness and hope that this story brings, there were also times of unyielding pain and indescribable sorrow. Cancer is something that affects every aspect of a person's life—physical, social, emotional, spiritual; nothing is safe. Likewise, it reaches out and engulfs the family as well, stripping them to reveal the very core of who they are and what they are made of. When faced with this disease, a person and his or her family have the choice to withdraw inward, to focus on their own hurt and pain, to become prey long before the cancer takes any physical toll. On the other hand, they can choose to rise above, to not sink, to stand steadfast hand in hand as the storm rages on around them. A family can choose to reach out and rescue one another as they strive to carry each other's heartache.

I would never pretend that there is a one-size-fits-all approach to cancer. Just as every case and physical treatment vary based on the individual, so it goes with the emotional response that every person and family must have. As for our family, we knew that we needed to stay as close to each other as possible. We knew that if we could fully rely on each other, there was no force on earth that could overtake

1

us. However, we also recognized that our strength alone would not be enough.

I can't say that our lives have been easy. Likewise, I can't say that our lives have been hard. It would suffice me to say that our lives have been a journey, one that has allowed us to learn and to grow—a journey that took us places that we never would've dared venture, challenged us to the very heart of who we were, and allowed us the opportunity to learn more absolutely, love more completely, and live more fully.

First, a little background on our family: Kris and I married young and knew we wanted to start a family right away. A week before our first anniversary, we found out we were expecting Alexis. Cameron followed just a few years later, and then Olivia and Aleah were not far behind. We were a typical family who truly loved spending time together. We loved the outdoors, all sporting events (we consider dance a sport in our house), and just laughing together. If it is important to one of us, it is important to all of us, so the majority of any and all free time was pretty much spent together. We had our challenges, but we always had a roof over our heads (albeit a leaky one at one point) and food to eat. We lived in an old community rich in tradition and rocky soil—our diamond in the rough. We contentedly lived each day with no knowledge of the monster that was preparing to strike our little family.

Second, a little personal insight into my psyche: I am a person who loves to learn, and I truly believe that each situation we find ourselves in allows us a unique opportunity to learn and grow. Throughout the course of this experience, I have learned things that I know I would not have learned in any other setting. My heart has been completely broken, reconstructed, shattered, and then built again more times than I can count as I witnessed my child hit and smash through what I had previously deemed a physical rock bottom. I know that no parent would allow their child to suffer without reason, so rather than focus on what we were going through, I tried to think of why we were going through it and what was to be learned.

This was not because of some inner strength I possessed but a necessity I adopted to cope and process the unthinkable circumstances we found ourselves in. Due to the sensitive nature of this experience, I share it with permission and encouragement from Kris and my children in hopes that it may offer peace, comfort, or understanding for someone else who may be experiencing trials in his or her life. This story is one that is based on faith, love, and one of the only choices that wasn't taken from us—the choice to be happy.

Chapter One

Let This Cup Pass from Us
(Luke 22:42)

The sky was dark as thunderclouds threatened to keep the promise of rain that hung in the air. But it wasn't the darkness that caught my eye; it was the rays of light that could not be withheld by the gloom surrounding them. I was driving to work, still looking to develop some sort of normalcy for the first time in two years.

I pondered on the beauty of the beams of light breaking through the darkest of billows and the majesty it seemed to hold. I wondered why the sun didn't always capture my attention the way it did on that day. Slowly, I realized it was not the sun that changed, but my awareness and need of it. On warm, bright days, I assumed the sun was there without ever looking up and fully appreciating it. It was not until the clouds rolled in and the storm started that I began to actively search for the sun, needing the reassurance that it had not forsaken me.

I continued my drive as my mind reluctantly wandered over the events of the past two years—proceedings I still could not yet fully grasp had taken place, trials I struggled to believe my family had endured. Images and emotions accompanied vivid flashbacks of memories that were forever etched into the very fabric of my being. Some I would forever cherish; others still made it hard to sleep at night. There were good days, great days, and hard days. And then there were days that were too difficult to relive, revisit, and at times fully comprehend. My thoughts delved further than usual, and I allowed them to continue, not having the emotional strength to stop them that day.

As I pulled into the parking lot, I glanced back to the sky. The shadows continued to grow—a serious storm was inevitable—yet the beams of light continued to shine in defiant contrast. I felt the corners of my mouth involuntarily turn slightly upward into a melancholy smile as the memories took over.

September 11 is a notable day for many people. In 2015, it became forever etched in our hearts for a different reason.

"Honey, how's your back this morning? Did you even sleep last night?" I asked our oldest daughter, Alexis, as she groggily packed what she would need for school that day. It was homecoming week at her high school, and her drill team had been holding an increased number of practices in order to prepare for their upcoming performances. Although she was only a sophomore, this was her second year on the team, but for some reason, her body seemed to be struggling more already this season than it had even a few months earlier.

"Not really," she said sleepily while moving with more effort than normal. "I've tried heat packs, ibuprofen, Tylenol—everything. Nothing is helping. I'm in so much pain, Mama. I don't know what is going on."

My brow furrowed as I looked at her makeshift bed on the couch. She had opted to sleep there the night before, thinking that by sleeping in a more upright position she may be able to relieve some of the pressure and pain that was causing her so much discomfort.

"Let me look at your back again, Lex." She paused her packing momentarily to point out the tenderest parts and mentioned that the pain extended into her abdomen as well. To my surprise, I noticed that she appeared to be more swollen than she had the day before. Would a pulled muscle really swell like that?

"We need to get going," Lexi said, breaking my concentration. "If I'm late, I can't perform at the assembly today."

"Okay," I said, still lost in thought. "Lex, are you sure you feel good enough for school today? Maybe you should stay home and rest. You didn't sleep at all last night, and I think I need to take you to the doctor."

"No, I need to go or I can't perform. I'll rest after school. I can have the trainer look at it if you're worried. I'll be good, Mama." We walked to the car and drove to the school. I noticed as she walked into school that she seemed to be moving slower than normal. Perhaps it was just the extra practices, the added routines, or the push to accomplish new goals, but it felt like more than that. Lexi had never been a morning person, but this was more than just exhaustion.

A few short hours later, I was back at the school for the assembly and the drill team's first of three performances for the day. As the assembly commenced, I found a spot to stand among the other drill moms. A familiar voice came over the loudspeaker. "Please welcome your world-famous Cyprus High Spinnakers!" The crowd applauded boisterously as the girls took the floor in perfect unison. They came to their starting positions and held tightly despite the catcalls until the music began. My eyes quickly found Lexi, as they always did when she danced. Her long, slender frame was easy to pick out. As I watched her perform the hip-hop routine, I unknowingly bit my lower lip and knew without a doubt that something was very wrong. The pain on her face was evident—even when she danced.

Immediately following the assembly, I checked Lexi out of school to let her recover at home. After her rest she returned to school, determined to attend an extra practice for the two routines her team would perform that night. She came home after the practice and got ready for yet another performance while counting down the minutes until she could have some more medication, in the futile hope it might take the edge off. By now the pain she was describing was indicative of appendicitis. Her back had a deep ache, and her abdomen had a sharp, stabbing pain. With the amount of tenderness she exhibited, I began to fear that her appendix had ruptured.

"Lex, I really need to take you to the emergency room," I said while simultaneously playing Dr. Mom and checking for a fever. "If your appendix has burst, it is extremely dangerous, and you could need an operation tonight." She continued packing for her upcoming performance, and we continued our conversation on the way to her school.

"I just need to wait until after our performances, Mom. We've already cleaned the dances, and if I don't go out there, the spacing will be off. Besides, I saw the trainer, and she said she thinks the pain and swelling is just a muscle spasm, so I should just rest this weekend and go to the doctor if it is still bothering me on Monday."

"It might be nothing," I replied, "but I will feel much better after we know for sure that it is nothing. Did the trainer tell you it was okay to still perform?" The car came to a stop as I glanced over at Lexi.

She didn't quite meet my eyes. "Well . . . not exactly. She said it would be in my best interest to sit this one out just in case, but it's homecoming, Mom, and I need to do this for my team." She hurried on as she exited the car. I followed suit, knowing full well that her mind was already set. "We've all worked so hard. Besides, I said a prayer and asked Heavenly Father to help me be able to perform to the best of my ability. I will be okay to dance. I know it."

We had made it to the football field, where her team would perform. The conversation had trailed off, and I turned to glance at my daughter. The look in her eyes told me that this was a battle that would not be easily won, and her pure yet simple faith put my heart at ease for the moment. I kissed her cheek and she joined her team. I watched as they took the field, and then I quickly made my way back to the opposite side of the field. Kris and the kids had driven over separately to save us seats, and I quickly found them. As a family we watched her perform like we had so many times before, but this time there was a feeling of uneasiness in the pit of my stomach that would not subside. Every count of eight seemed to drag on, and although the performance was flawless, it could not have ended soon enough. While watching her dance, Kris and I decided that as soon as she was off the field I would take her to the hospital.

The music had not yet quit playing as I kissed Kris and the kids good-bye and made my way around the track to where the girls would exit the field. I met Lexi at the gate and put my arm around her. She was weaker than she had been twenty minutes before. She smiled and told her friends good-bye while simultaneously leaning heavily on me and trying not to draw attention to herself. The farther we walked, the more evident it became that she could no longer bear her own weight. "Mom, what if I have to have surgery to remove my appendix? Will I have to stay in the hospital long? Do you think there is still a chance I can go to the dance with my friends tomorrow? I really can't miss practice on Monday."

We headed to the dance room to collect her bags. I answered her questions and calmed her fears the best I could while helping her into the car. We began the twenty-minute trek to Primary Children's Hospital, and I drove as quickly and gently as I could. With every turn and slight bump in the road, I could see my daughter tense and wince from the pain. She rode hunched over, grasping at her stomach. My heart ached for her. There were so many times over the years that I had watched her gracefully perform while bruised and broken without the slightest indication that she was even in pain, so for her to exude such symptoms terrified me. Something was horribly wrong.

I parked the car as quickly as I could and exited the vehicle. Lex gingerly stepped out of the car and asked if she could hold on to my arm to help steady herself while she walked. This wasn't right. My independent daughter who never wanted any additional attention was asking to lean on me and for me to walk slower. Each step was heavy with effort. One of her arms was around my neck and the other around her stomach. My mind was racing. What was happening inside her body that could cause such drastic changes so quickly?

We entered the emergency room with Lexi still decked out in her performance attire—looking entirely too dolled up to be among the sea of sick children. We checked in and took our place among them. Her red lipstick and glittered eyelids did not exactly scream emergency. Upon entry they asked what symptoms Lex was having.

Apparently what she described combined with her appearance was not enough to necessitate an emergency, so we were left to wait.

Everyone processes pain differently. For Lexi, she found a tolerable position, sat very still, and remained very quiet. She maintained her poise and manner, making her suffering nearly undetectable to someone who did not know her. However, the intensity of the hurt she was in was visible in her blue eyes, and it made me ache for her. The pain continued to worsen. At this point, I was hoping Lexi would begin running a fever, screaming out, or doing something that was significant enough for them to move faster and treat this with more urgency. I saw her wince yet again as the muscles in her jaw clenched and her grip on her stomach tightened.

"Sis, can you start throwing a fit or something so they will know how much pain you're actually in? I know it's not your style to bring attention to yourself, but I hate seeing you hurting like this. I just want them to get you back there so we can get some answers."

She gave me a tender smile. "I don't like to show people how much pain I'm really in or complain about it a lot. It doesn't really change anything, and it just makes people worry. So, if you think about it, it doesn't really accomplish anything." I kissed her head as she slowly leaned it back down on my shoulder.

Time moves at a slower pace when your child is in pain, and it felt like an eternity had passed. "Alexis Gould." I'd never been so grateful to an ER tech for calling out a name. She checked us in, and we were escorted to what would be our private room for the next fourteen hours. As procedure goes, the tech came in, then the nurse, and finally the doctor entered the room and examined her. He noticed the extreme sensitivity in her abdomen and back and ordered an ultrasound. "Do you have any questions for me before I have them take you back, Lexi?"

With a sheepish grin, she replied, "Is there any way I can eat something yet? I'm really hungry, and they said I have to ask you first." I smiled. Nothing seemed to impact my daughter's healthy appetite.

"Not yet," the doctor replied. "Just in case surgery does need to be done. Let's get some imaging done." Then, seeing the look of disappointment on Lexi's face, he added, "But I promise that as soon as I know for sure that it is safe, I'll let you eat." This was enough to get a smile out of her, which in turn drew a smile from the doctor.

The ultrasound was done, and we were taken back to our room. I was certain it would be at least another hour before we saw anyone for results, but within twenty minutes we had a new technician that was in and out of our room so constantly I was certain she must be assigned to just Lex. A nurse also came in and said that they were going to start Lexi on a morphine drip to help with the pain and needed to hook her up to consistent monitors. My worn-out brain figured they had discovered that it was appendicitis and that she actually was in a great deal of pain.

A short time later, the doctor re-entered only to report that they had been unable to find the elusive appendix and that they would like to do more imaging. "We need to do an X-ray and possibly a CT scan and an MRI." I nodded in fatigued agreement, thinking to myself that for a body part that is said to have no vital function, this appendix was proving to be extremely problematic.

"Do you have any questions for me?" the doctor asked Lexi.

She exhaled slowly and with a melancholy smile said, "This means I'm going to have to wait a little longer before I get my nachos, huh?" He nodded his head apologetically, and with much effort, she repositioned herself to where she was comfortable once again and allowed the morphine to get back to work as she drifted to sleep.

I'm fairly certain that the chairs in the emergency room are designed to make you want to leave so they can weed out who really needs to be there and who is just overreacting to their child's bee sting. My body was shifting from a growing unease to exhaustion and back again. I waited as patiently as one can wait in the unforgiving chair. The hours were passed trying to distract myself by alternating between texting Kris any inkling of an update and trying to beat my high score at 1010. Techs came to check vitals and take

Lexi from one imaging appointment to another, and nurses came to adjust the flow of medication. Lexi caught me unsuccessfully trying to get comfortable and offered to switch between the bed and the chair with me. I thanked her and declined, grateful that the morphine seemed to be controlling the pain enough that she was finally able to get intermittent rest.

A new doctor wearing green scrubs entered the room. I would later learn that the color of his scrubs meant that he was a surgeon. As he scrolled through various images on the computer screen, he told us that the results from the ultrasound and the CT scan had come back. He finally arrived at what he thought was a clear enough image for my non-medical brain to process and began pointing things out. "This here is the stomach. This is the liver. This is her pancreas, and there are intestines here. This area," he said as he circled a large kidney-bean shape that seemed to be crowding everything else in the abdomen, "is an abnormal mass that we believe is malignant."

Upon hearing those words, a parent's mind goes blank. Logically you know what malignant means, but emotionally you cannot process it.

The surgeon continued. "We will need to biopsy this mass to make that final determination." He left me alone with my sleeping child and a stream of endless questions I did not want to ask.

I looked over to see that the effects of the morphine were still letting Lexi rest, and then I quietly stepped out of the room to call Kris. I needed him. I needed his voice. I needed to not hear what I had just been told. This was not news that could be texted. I took some deep breaths and tried to hide the terror in my voice. He answered after just one ring. "Hey babe, have they found out what's going on yet?"

I inhaled and slowly exhaled, and in the calmest voice I could muster, I replied, "Uh, so they are saying that she has a large abnormal mass in her abdomen." There was silence as the words crept through the phone line.

"Wait, what? So what does that mean? What are they going to do? Does she need surgery to remove it then? When are they going to take it out?"

I continued to reiterate the few details I had. "They are going to keep her here until they can do a biopsy on Monday morning. They think it may be malignant . . ." The words rushed out now. Any sense of composure I had escaped along with that last word. "They think she has cancer. How can she have cancer? She hasn't even been sick for long. Should I have brought her in sooner? How did I miss this? She can't have cancer—can she?"

I could sense Kris trying to breathe steadily as he spoke, the tide shifting as his calmness now tried to balance out my emotions. "Everything is going to be okay, babe. Just take a breath. They are just being overly cautious. I'll head up now and give her a blessing. Just breathe, honey. It will be okay."

By this time it was early Saturday morning and the dawning of a new day in our lives. Word had begun to spread about the results of the imaging. Dear friends and family sent us message after message, telling us not to worry, that the mass would be nothing, and my mind wanted to believe them. But in my heart I knew that our lives would never be the same.

Kris arrived at the hospital, and I met him just outside Lexi's ER room. My worn-out body collapsed into his strong embrace. Few words were spoken—none were needed. He entered the room and walked over to Lexi's bed. Lovingly he rubbed her head. "Hey, Lexi-girl."

Still under the effects of the morphine, she groggily opened her eyes and smiled up at him. "Hey, Dad-o," she said. He returned the smile, loving that she still referred to him by the first name she ever called him. Our time was limited since they were preparing to transfer Lexi to a more permanent room, but our hearts knew we needed to hear what God had in store for our daughter. Humbly Kris placed his hands on Lexi's head, and with the power and authority of the priesthood of God, he gave her a blessing. It was very specific and talked about how she would be fully healed and that her body would once again return to doing the things she loved to do. This was not the end of her life, but the beginning. Lexi listened intently to the words spoken to her through the power of the priesthood. They gave her a sense of peace and strength in knowing that whatever was to come, she would get through it.

We were transferred from the emergency room to a room on the fourth floor—the ICS (Immuno-Compromised Service)—the cancer floor. Parts of the floor were being remodeled, and sheetrock had been put up to minimize the effects of the dust and debris from the construction. A few boxes of markers were attached to the wall, encouraging those who passed to decorate the otherwise boring hallway. We passed walls that were artfully designed with words of strength and hope for the tiny warriors who currently or had previously occupied these rooms.

My eyes fell on the words "You've got this!" and "Never, ever give up!" It was all I could do to read them, let alone process them. I glazed over many other messages, much like the rest. Toward the end of the makeshift wall, about three feet up, in a perfect, small-child font were printed the words "No one fights alone." A warmth washed over me. I had not yet reached a place of feeling that I was ready for battle, but I had already felt the comfort of knowing that whatever lie ahead, we would not be facing it alone.

My mind was reeling. I still couldn't comprehend why we were being taken to the cancer unit. In my ignorance to the knowledge that cancer is no respecter of persons, I just kept thinking, *They are making a mistake. Cancer does not run in our family, and Lexi hasn't even been that sick. This just doesn't make any sense.*

A set of double doors opened with the push of a button, only to present another set. There was a sign after the first set of doors instructing patrons that everyone wishing to enter must wash and sanitize their hands. We washed, sanitized, and walked into the unit. We were led to the third room on the right. A bottle of sanitizer with a friendly reminder to sanitize before entering the room was attached to the outside of the door. I've always been a big hand-washer, but this seemed a little much. We obliged, and as I was rubbing my already-clean hands with more sanitizer, I noticed that the door next to ours had been fully decked out with numerous decorations. The blinds on the door's window were pulled up, and I couldn't help but glance in. The room looked exciting–jubilant even! Posters, decorations, and knickknacks were in full bloom. The fun atmosphere of the room felt out of place with the heavy emotions I was carrying in my heart. It occurred to me that people could be in the hospital and have fun. This seemed like a foreign concept.

I numbly followed as they wheeled our daughter into the room she would be staying in until the biopsy was done and we could return home. I was aware of Kris's hand in mine, like it had been a thousand times before, but it was as if his hand was the only thing keeping me grounded to reality. We chatted with caring nurses who greeted us warmly, and I tried to smile and make small talk. I could hear what I knew to be my voice answering questions but felt as if my body was a shell of what it had been just twenty-four hours prior. On the outside I was trying to smile, trying to mask the fear that had been dropped on me when the word "malignant" had been spoken by the surgeon, but on the inside I felt hollow, like nothing would ever be okay again.

We crossed the threshold into our small room. It was large enough for a hospital bed, a couch that doubled as a cot, and a rocking chair. The back wall sported a sink that was reachable when sitting on the cot, and the door to the bathroom was right behind the sink. I was impressed to learn that the bathroom did come with its own shower, but I soon realized that any convenience with having a private bathroom extended no farther than the patient. Due to the close monitoring of the patients and the hazardous nature of the medications given to them, no one except the patient was allowed to use the facilities inside the room.

The room was painted a light taupe, with one accent wall a calming blue. I imagined that someone somewhere had done research and found that these particular colors would help nurture a sense of peace and general calmness. It wasn't having this effect on me. A whiteboard had been decorated with the words "Welcome to ICS, Alexis!" The room was much more comfortable than the emergency room we had previously occupied, and we were grateful—exhausted, but grateful. However, despite all the efforts to make the room comfortable and welcoming, it was still very clear that functionality had triumphed over feng shui in the layout and design of our new habitat.

Our nurse came in and introduced herself. She must have noticed the blank looks on our faces, as I'm sure she had seen multiple times before. Rather than ask certain questions about things we couldn't answer, she went right to work making sure that Lexi was comfortable. I could feel the love with which she cared for Lex, even though she had just met her. I quickly learned that it took a distinct personality to work on this floor. You had to have the ability to see the worst life had to offer and yet continue to hope for the best. It was a trait I was determined to adopt.

While Lexi was getting settled, one of the techs occupied Kris and me by giving us the official tour of the ICS floor and all the amenities it had to offer. The first thing we learned was that we had been given prime real estate—there was a restroom located just a few doors down from our room. The ICS floor is divided into four pods, each one having a series of rooms on either side of the hall. The air in the room is pressurized and filtered. If a door is left open, an alarm sounds, reminding the staff and the occupants that the door needs to remain closed. Every door has a two- by three-foot window in the middle. The patients can choose to open the blinds to the window on their door and look out into the hall or keep them closed to offer a false sense of privacy. We walked past numerous open windows and saw children of all ages inside. They all shared one prominent characteristic—there was not a full head of hair in sight.

We were brought to the "parent lounge." This too was built for functionality. It was a kitchen, laundry room, and bathroom all rolled into about fifty square feet. The door opened, and immediately we passed another door on our right. This led to a restroom. We continued three feet to a counter on the right and a common fridge directly in front of us that held meals and drinks for everyone on the ICS floor. The counter had a sink, coffee maker, and toaster oven. Above the counter were a few cupboards with paper plates and a small assortment of snack items. Just to the left were two stackable washer/dryer combos. A small counter opposite them held the microwave, as well as the laundry detergent and dryer sheets. We were instructed that anything going into the fridge needed to be labeled with the patient's name and room number, and when we did our laundry, that same information would need to be written on the page attached to each machine. On our way back, we were shown the one shower on the floor. A toilet was in there as well, making a total of three on the floor that were for parent use.

We made it back to our room, and Kris suggested that I take a minute to shower. It had been an incredibly long night, and I hadn't yet eaten (because Lexi couldn't). He reminded me that nothing of note was scheduled to happen for a few days. I collected the few toiletries he had brought for me and headed to the shower. Luckily, I found it without getting lost, and luckier still, it was open. I found myself alone for the first time in what seemed like eternity. Everything was different, and I knew it. I could finally allow myself to feel it. I'm not sure if my tears or the shower accounted for more water, but either way, I felt better once I got out.

I looked around, but I couldn't find where the clean towels were kept. There were no cupboards in there, no places that towels could be hiding. This room was even more basic than the others. It had only a toilet, a shower, a sink, a garbage can, and a hamper. Nothing else. My mind went back to the tour—where had the nurse said that the towels were? I realized she hadn't said. I had just assumed that they would be next to the shower, like the laundry soap was next to the washer. However, that was not the case.

I finally accepted the fact that there I stood, completely dripping wet. My only options for resolving this dilemma were a wall blow-dryer that looked older than I was, a hamper full of strangers' used towels, and the paper towel dispenser that looked as if it had recently been stocked. Oddly, this was not the most exposed I had felt in the past twenty-four hours. With a renewed energy brought on by my recent breakdown, I simply shrugged my shoulders, thought to myself, *This is not the hardest thing I've had to do today*, and went to work drying off with paper towels. It provided us with a much-needed laugh when I went back to our room to reiterate the details of my dilemma.

Chapter Two

We Will Not All Sleep, but We Will All Be Changed

(1 Corinthians 15:51)

The next few days passed without my knowing. I'm sure that the sun rose and set and that people ate, laughed, and slept, but I did none of those things. I did the only thing I had the emotional energy to do—I waited. I waited to learn the fate of my family—of my child. During the day I greeted visitors. I thanked them for their thoughts and prayers and did my best to restate the events that had led us there. During the night I sat and listened to my daughter breathe. I tried to relax to the humming of the monitors that she was now connected to, or walked numbly through the empty hallways of the hospital with the echo of my solitary footsteps as my only companion.

One visit in particular will forever replay in my mind. Primary Children's Hospital is home to some of the best people you never want to meet. One of the technicians that had cared for Lexi in the ER, the one who seemed to be caring solely for Lex once the imaging was done, took time after her shift to visit us once we were settled in our room. She brought Lex a small statue that symbolized courage and told her to always remember that while the doctors were very intelligent, ultimately they were not the ones in charge. "Remember that miracles are real, and even when the odds are not in your favor, the seemingly impossible can happen," she said.

She expressed her love and encouragement and left our room. I was grateful for the visit and tried to brush it off as caring—though slightly extreme advice—since we didn't know if Lex even had cancer. She clearly knew more than I was willing to admit.

The day I had been simultaneously dreading and anticipating—the day of the biopsy—had arrived, and Lexi was taken into surgery. I wanted to believe that after this procedure we could all go home knowing that Lexi didn't have cancer, that this was just a terrible mistake that had somehow been blown way out of proportion. I wanted to be the mom who was overreacting to the bee sting. I wanted to leave the cancer floor and never need to use the parent shower or label my own food again. But my heart was being prepared for what my head was still trying to dismiss.

The surgeon completed the biopsy and called Kris and me back to the consultation room. We walked behind him hand in hand and sat down as he closed the door. He began speaking, but the only thing I heard was that word again. *Malignant.* I knew what it meant, but my only response was, "So you're saying that my daughter has cancer?" Kris's hand tightened around mine. My jaw clenched to keep a sob from escaping. The doctor continued, saying that the tumor presented as lymphoma, but that further pathology would be completed to verify the type of cancer and formulate a specific treatment plan.

"We also found that Lexi's tumor had ruptured," the doctor continued. "That was likely the cause of the sudden onset of intense pain. She also needed a blood transfusion. Overall, she is doing well. She is in recovery now. Once they are ready, they will find you in the waiting room. Do you have any questions for me?"

I did, but I didn't want to hear the answers. In our family's former, healthy life, I would have been terrified that my child was sick enough to need a blood transfusion. In this life, I was quickly learning that there were greater horrors out there. We thanked him for his time and numbly walked hand in hand back to the waiting room. Kris spoke to our family, who had anxiously been waiting to hear the news, while I held tighter to his hand. Tears were shed and embraces given, but it was as if I could feel none of it. I was simply observing the situation without experiencing it.

We were then taken to the recovery room. The nurses attending to Lexi were smiling and saying that she had been asking for us and telling them all about how in love we were. We reached her bedside, and she asked for each of our hands. She sleepily said she would never let them go. I smiled and responded to her words, but my mind was reeling. How would we tell her that she had cancer? How do you tell a child—*your* child—that she has cancer? I knew one thing for sure. I wanted to tell her in a private setting, one where she could cry, or scream, or tell us how unfair it was, because I was feeling all of those things.

We continued to make small talk with her as she held onto our hands. This was the first surgery she had ever had, and the anesthetic proved to be quite a truth serum. We laughed as she candidly told us stories intertwined with her honest yet tactless opinions. If our hands ever adjusted, she would ask us to immediately put them back. She said again that she wanted to hold our hands forever and never let them go. I decided then that this promise was one that I would hold her to.

Lex was now stable enough that she could return to her room. We silently followed the nurse as she pushed Lexi's bed back to the fourth floor—ICS—the cancer floor. Only now we really belonged there. We would have to find a way to fight this, to never, ever give up. We passed a nurse that knew we were having the biopsy that day. "Hey! How did things go?" she asked.

"She has cancer. They said it looks like lymphoma," I solemnly replied.

To my surprise, the nurse smiled. "Lymphoma? That's great!"

I was stunned, to say the least. Perhaps she didn't hear what I had said—my child had cancer. This meant that there was something in her body trying to kill her, something that had already claimed too many victims, and it was just confirmed that she had it. Where was the excitement in that? I soon found out.

Kris and I continued walking behind Lexi's bed and stood numbly as her nurse got her settled once again in her room. We held her hand and began to explain the results of the biopsy. We looked in her eyes and said aloud the words that no parent should ever have to utter to their child. "Lex, you have cancer." It felt surreal. This couldn't be happening. I expected to see a flash of hurt or anger, but there was only surprise—shock. The words had barely escaped our lips when an oncologist entered the room.

She stood by Lexi's bedside and explained to her that while no cancer is considered good, there are definitely cancers that are less aggressive and more treatable than others. Given the localization of the tumor, lymphoma was one of those in this case. I hadn't considered the fact that there was an upside to having a certain cancer in a certain case, but there was.

As the oncologist stood by her bed and explained to Lexi how curable lymphoma was given these circumstances, and that she fully expected her to grow to be a little old lady, my heartbeat slowed a little. This was the silver lining we had so desperately needed to hear. Yes, our child had cancer, but in this case, they were confident she could be completely cured. Given the locality of the tumor, they were very optimistic. The doctor's demeanor offered so much hope that I felt the weight ease off our shoulders. This would be a difficult journey, but it was one that could be won.

Lexi spent the next few hours processing the news she had just received.

"How are you doing, honey?" I asked her.

"It doesn't feel real, Mama. It feels like someone else's life. I was just at school dancing. We were just camping and hiking. I just don't feel like I have cancer."

Cam, Liv, and Leah came to the hospital so we could be together in person when our children found out. We needed them to be able to ask us any questions, voice any concerns, and shed any tears together. The six of us sat together, each of our kids taking turns climbing into Lexi's hospital bed to cuddle with her and cuddling up next to us.

We talked about the success rate of lymphoma and how curable Lexi's case would be. We talked about how she would likely lose her hair and that we would have to make some life changes for the next few months. We talked about how we would likely feel many emotions during this journey and that it was okay to feel them. We talked about the reality that people do lose their lives to cancer, but reaffirmed the blessing that Lexi had been given and asked each of our children to hold tightly to that blessing. It was a hard yet hopeful day, and we felt blessed despite our circumstances.

Visitors continued to come to show their love and support. Among them, our stake presidency came to visit. At their hands and through the power of God, Lexi received another blessing. Again, she was reminded in very clear terms that this was not the end of her mortal life, but the beginning. Those words meant more this time with the news we had received earlier that day. She was reminded that this experience would prepare her to be able to fulfill her mission here on earth. Somehow Lexi knew that this was what she had to go through to be who Heavenly Father needed her to be, and she humbly told me she would do it.

I realized that throughout my life I had vowed many times to do what Heavenly Father asked of me. Many times I had thought how I would react to situations or how I would handle the trials I had to go through in my life. Like others, I had offered my will to Heavenly Father, knowing that He could make more of me than I could ever make of myself. However, watching your child take that same road when you don't feel strong enough to travel it with her is an extremely humbling experience. We had strived to prepare our children for the trials they would face, but how was she so prepared to handle this when I was not?

The following morning, five oncologists entered our room and greeted Lexi, Kris, and me. They had each brought their own chairs and sat in a line at the foot of Lexi's bed. Lexi was sitting in her bed, and Kris and I were sitting hand in hand on the cot that now doubled as my bed. My mind assumed that this was the official "you have cancer" visit and that they would outline the treatment plan and fill us in on the precautions we would need to take in order to keep Lex safe during this time.

The oncologist who had spoken with us the night before was there, and I noticed that her face appeared much more somber than it had the previous day. If I didn't know better, I would've thought that they were coming to deliver bad news, but surely she had told them that we already knew Lex had cancer. After all, what news could they give us that was worse than hearing "Your child has cancer"? Little did we know that what we thought was the silver lining in our clouds was actually lightening preparing to strike our family.

The doctors began to speak and told us that further testing had come back. They said that what had originally presented as lymphoma was actually neuroblastoma—cancer of the nerves. This team of oncologists told us that the pathology of the tumor had come back as unfavorable, and that Lexi had officially been diagnosed as having high-risk neuroblastoma. This is the most aggressive form of neuroblastoma, the kind that has a 30 percent survival rate and a recurrence rate of 55 percent. They said that her case was very unique. According to statistics, approximately 650 children in the United States are diagnosed with neuroblastoma every year. Of those, only 2 percent are diagnosed over the age of ten.

Kris then asked the only "cancer question" he ever asked. "Since this is a little kid cancer and Lexi is older and her nervous system has had more time to develop, does that increase the likelihood she will beat it?"

They met our gaze solemnly and ever so slightly shook their heads. "The older a person is when diagnosed, the more aggressive this cancer is." With somberness in their eyes, they continued, "Lexi is the oldest patient by four years that we have ever treated with this type of cancer."

My world was spinning. I found myself praying for her to have lymphoma. Who would've ever thought that a person would pray for their child to have lymphoma?! But I did! I wanted her to have the cancer that was highly curable in her case; the one that only required one doctor to break the news; the one that would all but guarantee her a full recovery and a long life. However, that was not the road we were meant to travel.

I couldn't bear to look at Kris. I didn't need to. I could feel the pain of his heart breaking by the hold he had on my hand. I ventured a glance at Lex, and to my surprise, I saw no fear, no anger—just her jaw clenched in pure determination. Perhaps she did not understand the statistics we were given. Maybe she had decided to zone out so she did not have to listen to the reality that was now part of her fifteen-year-old world. I couldn't blame her if that was the case. I wished I could do the same thing.

The informal conference taking place in our hospital room continued on. An aggressive cancer required aggressive treatment. We were told that Lexi's treatment would consist of six rounds of inpatient chemotherapy, a major surgery, a stem cell transplant, radiation, and then six rounds of antibody therapy. Upon completion, the doctors would re-evaluate to give us further instructions on how to proceed. There was no "After this you will be in remission and life can resume as normal." Their exact words were, "We are going to throw everything that we have at this and go from there."

On the outside I appeared composed, but something in my head was screaming. This was a mistake. There must have been some mistake. This couldn't be real. Our daughter was healthy and living a typical teenage life. Just days ago her biggest concern was deciding whether to highlight her hair or not, and now she was told that there was something growing inside of her, threatening her life?!

We were given information on how to proceed once we were home, what signs to look for, and when to call the doctor. The information was overwhelming—how high is too high for a fever, how long is too long for a nosebleed, what signs are indicative that your child needs a transfusion. The biggest thing that was emphasized was the importance of protecting a child at all costs from sickness during chemo. I knew enough about chemo to know that it weakened a person's immune system. What I didn't realize is that it does not just weaken the immune system. It makes it completely nonexistent.

Many people believe in exposing their children to different minor illnesses in hopes of naturally boosting their immune system. This was never my particular style, but I also wasn't the kind of person who went despondent when my child came in contact with someone who had a cold. I soon realized, however, that I was about to be. There is a switch that gets flipped when a doctor looks you directly in the eye and tells you, "To others it may be just a cold, but we have lost children to colds." He paused. "Your child can die from a cold." Nothing drives a point home like your child's life hanging in the balance. It was then that I realized that I was about to become the sanitizing mom. I would be the anti-germ, Lysol-loving, over-sanitizing mom. I had no other choice.

Luckily, all of the information they reviewed with us had been compiled into a handy binder. They must've learned that although the parents of newly diagnosed patients may nod their heads in acknowledgment, nothing is fully understood directly after hearing that your child has cancer. The binder sported a cartoon picture of a mom looking far too composed for me to relate to, pushing the wheelchair of a bald unisex child who had a very large smile on his or her face. We deemed it our "welcome-to-cancer binder" and planned to change the picture on the front as soon as we got home.

In a daze, we thanked the team of doctors for their time as they were leaving and turned to Lex to see how she was taking all of this. Less than twenty-four hours ago, she had been told that she had cancer, she would have to go through a few rounds of chemo, and she would likely lose her hair. She was told that it would be hard but that it was completely curable and within a few months she would be able to begin to return to her normal routine. Just as she was picking up the pieces from her world crashing down, a new bomb was dropped, causing her already crippled world to shatter.

It would no longer be enough for her to idly go through treatment. She would now have to actively fight for her life. She would endure what the doctors referred to as "highly intense treatment" that they would later re-evaluate to see how her body responded and then decide what she would need to do next.

The following days were spent being transported from our hospital room to appointments, meeting with specialists, completing baseline tests, and talking about the lasting effects of treatment—the price Lexi would have to pay to survive.

Losing her hair was minimal in comparison to the effects that this treatment would hold. She would likely lose some hearing, vision, organ function (if not complete organs themselves), and the ability to bear children. Ironically, the chemo that she would receive to cure her cancer could also potentially give her cancer. I shook my head at the cruel irony we faced. These side effects were tolerated only because there was no other option. This treatment had been proven to offer her the best chance at survival. The worst part was that after enduring all of this, there was less than a 30 percent chance that she would live.

I wanted to have faith, to believe. I wanted to be sure that Heavenly Father was aware that her situation was much more menacing than we had believed just twenty-four hours before. I wanted with my whole heart to completely crush any doubt that entered into my thoughts. My heart had the faith, but my head could only hear statistics as I tried to adapt to what was quickly becoming our new normal. A battle commenced between what I knew to be true and what I was being told. My exhausted body could not handle the inner turmoil I was facing.

I looked to Lexi, whose world had changed in an instant. I expected to see sadness or tears, frustration or anger. I was experiencing all of these emotions and thought that she must be as well. However, upon hearing side effect after side effect, Lexi set her jaw the way she had a million times before when she had decided to accomplish something.

We had just made it back to our room after completing the day's appointments.

"How are you doing, Lex?" I asked. "What are you thinking?"

She contemplated her answer before thoughtfully responding. "I know this will be difficult, but I know I can do it. Things happen for a reason, and if this is what I have to go through to become the person I am supposed to be, then I will do it. I'll be honest, Mom—I'm shocked I have cancer. I thought I was supposed to help the kids with cancer, not be the kid with cancer. A week ago I was dancing with my team. Now the doctors are telling me I might die. I know I won't, but I can tell that they don't know that yet. I'm not mad or angry. Cancer is going to take too much. It doesn't get to take my happiness. I'm just surprised, that's all."

"It's okay to be upset," I said, letting her know in these quiet moments that there was no need for her to be strong or hold anything in. "Your whole world just got rocked and flipped upside down. It's completely understandable."

"I'm really not mad. I'm sad that I might miss some performances, but God has a plan for me, and everything will be okay. He doesn't give us trials to be mean or because He hates us. He gives us trials because He loves us and wants us to grow and become stronger. I trust Him. I want to be dancing and going to school with my friends, but that is not what He needs me to be doing with my life right now. He needs me to be learning lessons by going through this trial. He needs me to make new friends at the hospital. He needs me to focus on strengthening my testimony, and I'll do whatever He needs me to do to become who He needs me to be." She jokingly added, "It would have been nice to have the less aggressive cancer, but because of the blessings I got, I know, without a doubt, that I will be okay."

Her faith was contagious, and I felt peace wash over me. I realized that she would be okay. She would have to endure horrors known only to a select few, but ultimately she would be okay. My feeble heart had no strength but to believe that the sacred promise she had been given would be kept. My peace was short lived however, when the thought of not just Lexi but also each of my kids and Kris came to my mind. Lexi would survive, this much we knew, but at what cost?

Cameron had just turned thirteen and had started the eighth grade. He had good friends, was making good choices, getting good grades, and honoring his priesthood. Olivia was ten and in the fifth grade. She was happy, loving life, and she thrived at being her own person. She excelled in school and lived care free. Aleah was almost eight years old. She would be getting baptized soon. She was in the third grade, and, like her siblings, she did well in school. She had lots of friends and loved to make people laugh. My children were far from perfect, but they were doing their best to make good choices. Up until this point, their lives were heading down distinct paths. Would those paths have to be sacrificed in order to save their sister?

Lexi's life was not the only one that had changed overnight. Cam, Liv, and Aleah would have to adjust from me taking them to and picking them up from school every day to me not being there at all on some days. They would have to learn that there would be times that, although we had made plans to do something as a family, things might have to be altered or rescheduled last minute to accommodate Lexi's nausea, fatigue, or sickness. They would have to stand by helplessly as they watched their sister, who used to jump on the trampoline with them, become too weak to walk herself to the car.

Change was inevitable. It always is. Trying to stop this change would be as likely as stopping a freight train with dental floss. As parents, Kris and I felt the full weight of the responsibility of making sure that their lives were altered in a positive way as we struggled to stay afloat in this sea of negativity.

Kris took the helm of life outside of the hospital. He began by meeting with the social worker at each of the kid's schools. He told them of the trial we were facing and signed any necessary paperwork for them to be able to speak to the social worker at any time they felt they needed to. We had always had open relationships with our children but recognized that we needed all of the additional resources we could get. We were dealing with emotions we had never encountered and didn't know where or when they might surface. We needed to be prepared on all fronts for whatever would arise. Cancer would not be Lexi's trial alone; we were all being challenged. Kris's days became divided between making sure that Lexi and I were okay and tending to the needs of Cam, Liv, and Leah. His heart had shattered, yet he remained a strength for us all—protecting any sense of normalcy in our home at all costs.

Chapter Three

Be Not Afraid

(Joshua 1:9)

*O*ur hearts were broken and our lives changed. This was a fact that we had to learn to live with. No amount of sadness or anger would change this. The only choice that remained was how we chose to live. At that exact moment, we had a decision to make. Did we truly believe what we had always claimed to believe? Did we really know there was a loving Father in Heaven who would keep the sacred promise that was given to Lexi through priesthood blessings? Did we understand that He had the capacity to love our children even more than we did and would help guide us to get them through this? Did we truly know that in the midst of our darkest trial He had indeed not forsaken us? Did we understand that when we cried out for Him in anguish He would really hear and answer us? Did we fully trust His plan, His timing, and ultimately His will? It is one thing to say these things aloud in a testimony meeting or a lesson, but we were being asked to fully live these principles in a way that we had never before been asked.

I couldn't breathe, I couldn't think, and at some point over the previous few days, my left leg had begun to involuntarily shake at inopportune times. My chest tightened, not from nerves or anxiety, but from pain. My heart was breaking. I had experienced heartache and sadness before, but this was different. I could feel a physical pain—a stabbing in my chest—from an emotional ache, an ache that I knew I couldn't fix. I knew that this was a pain reserved for emotional heartache that was much greater than my body could physically handle. It was in that moment that I realized that if I was going to survive, I would have to rely on someone much greater than myself. Someone who had also watched His child suffer in a way that I could not comprehend.

Out of habit I opened my scriptures, the way I had thousands of times before. I was searching for an immediate relief from my pain. My book fell open and my eyes immediately found Joshua 1:9: "Have not I commanded thee? Be strong and of a good courage; be not afraid neither be thou dismayed: for the Lord thy God is with thee whithersoever thou goest." I had found my respite. The pain I was feeling did not magically go away, but it became less suffocating. I could breathe again. I had been taught from the time I was little that Heavenly Father was always with me, that He would stay by my side as long as I wanted Him there. I had been shown evidences of this in my life time and time again, and we had taught our children the same thing. But as I read these words, I could now feel Him in a way I never had before. It was more than just a feeling; it was a presence. I was literally encircled in the arms of His love, and He held me as my heart sobbed.

I've always felt a closeness with my Father in Heaven, but my previous prayers paled in comparison to the ones I found myself offering. It wasn't that my prayers were any more or less sincere. The difference was that before I had felt like I had something to bring to the table. I could ask Heavenly Father for my needs, and in return I could serve or help someone else to show my gratitude. That was no longer the case. I was broken. I could only plead with Him to stay by our side, and in return I could offer only my trust in Him that when we needed Him most, He wouldn't leave us.

Over the course of the following days, we had visitor upon visitor coming to see Lexi. Our family, friends, and community and her teammates and coaches united as one. As a family, we were holding so tight to one another, and they surrounded us, making sure that even when we didn't have the strength to hold on, we couldn't let go. Gratitude filled my heart as I was told time and time again that we wouldn't be alone in this fight. We were completely sustained by loved ones during the day, but the nights were unbearable.

Sleep was a luxury reserved for another lifetime, and I wasn't sure that I would ever again reside there. Between the beeping of the monitors, the sound of the oxygen that was a recent addition to my daughter's new collection of tubes, and the nurses doing such a wonderful job of making sure that her vitals were consistently monitored, I became convinced that no one ever actually slept on this floor. Instead, I took to roaming the halls aimlessly with my thoughts as my only companion.

One night after Lexi had fallen asleep, I found myself out walking by the "crying couches." I had affectionately named them that because of a rule I had put in place, stating that no one could cry in Lexi's room except for her and her siblings. It was not that I was trying to mask the sadness; it was that Lexi was one who felt the need to constantly comfort and uplift those around her. As grateful as I was for this gift that she had, I wanted her to be able to feel her own emotions, on her own time, in her own way. I did not want her to feel the need to buoy up those around her when she felt she was sinking. On the other hand, when she was happy, I wanted to make sure that her room stayed as positive as possible. I held myself to this rule as well. So, on many occasions, I would go for a walk and find myself sobbing on the couches just outside of the ICS unit.

It was not quite a week into our journey, and I found myself having quite the pity party for Lex on one particular night, thinking of all the things that she would miss and all of the fun that typical teenagers were having. I found myself thinking how unfair it was that she only got to experience three short weeks of her sophomore year before she was diagnosed. I had made peace with the fact that this was the road that Lexi would need to travel. I knew she would survive, and if our mind-set was right, there was much we could learn from this experience.

However, the more I learned about what she would endure and the lasting effects of this treatment, the more I realized that even when Lexi was well enough to go back to her normal life, she would never again be a typical teenager. Again my heart sank. She should be focused on not breaking curfew and who her first kiss would be instead of whether she wanted to freeze her eggs to combat her likely infertility, or if she should cut her hair now or watch helplessly as it fell out. My head had made peace with this trial, but my heart was still bitter.

Luckily for me, Heavenly Father is extremely patient in His teachings. As I was walking and mourning the loss of this life, a question came into my mind. *What is it that you want more than anything for your children?*

Well, that answer was easy—I wanted them to become the people Heavenly Father wanted them to be.

Why?

Because I had seen enough of life to know that Heavenly Father knows much more than we do, and in order to be truly happy, we must follow His plan. I wanted my children to be truly happy in this life, and becoming who Heavenly Father wanted them to be was the most sure way to make that happen. They needed to understand that while they couldn't always control the situations life would give them, they could always control their response to those situations. By understanding their individual relationship with God, they would more fully be prepared to respond to whatever life had in store for them. Peace could be their companion even in times of strife.

Once that question had been answered, I again thought of the typical teenage experience, but this time I saw it through spiritual eyes. I thought of the teenage years that involve making decisions that affect the rest of a person's life. I thought of the life that comes with temptations and adversity. The life I would protect my child from if given the option. I thought of the realities of teenage life and what it could hold, not just the highlights. I was reminded that while Lexi may be missing out on performances and football games, she might also be being spared from situations that could ultimately damage her spirit. I silently thanked my Heavenly Father for this understanding and headed back to my room.

By the time I returned, Lexi was awake. She was still getting used to the chorus of beeps that the monitors made throughout the night, and she often struggled with the intensely of the vivid night terrors that were known to accompany some of her medications. When I returned, she decided to listen to a conference talk. We'd quickly learned that this practice calmed her and allowed her to peacefully put aside the terrors enough to get some rest. She had no idea of the struggle I had just had or the lesson I had just been taught, but as the talk began to play, I was humbled yet again.

Elder Von G. Keetch's calming voice filled our room as he told the story of a few young surfers who had traveled from America to Australia for the chance to surf some once-in-a-lifetime waves. To their dismay, when they arrived at the beach, they found that the area beyond the bay, the area where all of the best and biggest waves appeared to be, was sectioned off, making it impossible for them to surf there. They were frustrated and complaining about being held back by this seemingly useless barrier. It wasn't until a local surfer walked up to them and handed them a pair of binoculars that they were able to see the dorsal fins of large sharks that were feeding just beyond the barrier. The local man then reminded them to not be too critical about the barrier, for it was the only thing saving their lives.

This story solidified the lesson I had just learned. I had an idea of how high school would be for Lex, but I never saw this coming. I realized that this barrier, the one that I had seen as holding her back from "experiencing" high school, might actually be saving her life from unexpected dangers that I could not see. At times it is easy to see our trials as unnecessary stumbling blocks that hold us back from what we believe we are really supposed to be doing, but what if those trials are actually saving our lives in preparation for what is to come?

There are many things in this life that I do not know and have yet to understand. Yet as I watched my daughter drift to sleep amid the buzzing of monitors drowned out by the calming conference talk, I knew without a doubt that our Father in Heaven is aware of us.

Chapter Four

If Ye Are Prepared, Ye Shall Not Fear ·
(D&C 38:30)

I don't believe that anyone could be fully prepared for cancer. Nothing prepares you for the numbness in your limbs, the nausea in your stomach, or the physical pain that your heart feels upon hearing "Your child has cancer." Yet as I look back on this experience, I realize that while we might not have felt prepared to face cancer, we were absolutely prepared for the situations that would come about as a result of it.

For the three years before Lexi's diagnosis, Kris had been struggling with his own health problems. In March 2015, he was taken to an after-hours clinic because he was unable to breathe. An x-ray revealed that he had several large nodules filling up his chest. Multiple tests followed and revealed that his body had been functioning with just over 60 percent lung capacity. Testing continued, and lesser ailments were ruled out. We were told that at this point it could be one of only two things—lung cancer or sarcoidosis. A biopsy confirmed that it was indeed sarcoidosis (a disease in which benign nodules continue to multiply, filling up the lungs), and doctors told us that it was treatable with oral chemotherapy. These medications would attack his immune system and compromise his body in other ways. However, we felt relieved. We had come so close to cancer and managed to slip away. Regardless of how difficult the coming months of his treatment would be, we felt ourselves expressing gratitude to our Father in Heaven for sparing us from this trial.

It seems that when we are facing some of our greatest trials, we are able to more fully learn some of our most important lessons. Kris's treatment began wearing on him early on, and it was not having the effect the doctors had hoped it would. My heart hurt as I had to watch my best friend suffer with no sign of improvement. However, in the midst of my heartache and just weeks before Lexi was diagnosed, I was taught a very important lesson.

It was four in the morning, and I was waiting for the sun to rise on another day and chase away another sleepless night. My mind was replaying many scenarios, some that would come to pass and some that we'd be spared from. I looked around my home at the things that needed to be done, but I didn't have the emotional or physical strength to do them. I thought of the upcoming appointments, tests, and the schedules needing to be kept. I felt completely overwhelmed. I was gently reminded of a scripture I had just read that had quickly become one of my favorites: "For though I be absent in the flesh, yet am I with you in the spirit, joying and beholding your order, and the steadfastness of your faith in Christ" (Colossians 2:5).

Through these words I learned a few important truths. First, I was not alone and never had been. We all have fears and trials that we believe no one can fully understand, but we are not meant to bear these trials alone. Jesus Christ has experienced and overcome everything that any of us will ever have to experience. This was done willingly so that He would know exactly how to tend to our breaking hearts and aching souls with a perfectly unique understanding of our situation.

Second, I learned that it is okay to not be perfect. This scripture did not say that God finds joy in beholding my consistent perfection. If this were the case, I am afraid I would've never brought Him joy. Rather, it said that He finds joy in my order. At the time, my order might have looked like chaos to many, but it was the closest to order that I could find, and that was okay. It was okay that my laundry was not always done and that my poor flowerpots were a little crunchy.

Last, I learned that my trials would come and go, but the steadfastness of our faith would give us the strength we needed to endure those trials well and find true peace and happiness in our lives.

In addition to our family being prepared, Lexi had been individually prepared as well. Before her diagnosis, Lexi had made a special friend who would prove to play an extraordinary role in our lives. Lexi first met Lily when Lexi was twelve and Lily was two. They attended the same dance studio, and Lexi had been assigned to help Lily's class in the annual review. It took all of ten minutes for Lily to tell Lexi how much she loved her. From that moment on, they were best friends.

Over the coming years, the relationship continued to blossom. Lexi soon developed a relationship with Annika, Lily's little sister, as well. Annika was not quite a year old when Lexi first met Lily and the Rounds family. Annika had been diagnosed with neuroblastoma at only two months of age and had been fighting cancer almost her entire life. Lexi took note of the impact that cancer had on Lily and their family. She observed the love they had for one another, their closeness, their strength, and their happiness despite their trials. The more time Lexi spent with them, the more she had the desire to be a part of this world. She never dreamed that instead of a supporting role to those going through cancer, she would one day star in her own battle.

Months before discovering she had cancer, Lexi had spoken with Cheryl, Lily's mom, about the struggle that those going through cancer face. She had been working on her Young Women Personal Progress and wanted to base one of her projects on something that would benefit children who were fighting cancer.

"One of the most difficult things," Cheryl said, "is that chemo often makes the teenage girls and teenage boys look much the same. Treatments rob the youth of many physical characteristics that distinguish between young men and young women. As a result, young women have been mistaken for teenage boys, and that can be really damaging to their self-esteem."

This broke Lexi's heart. As a teenage girl herself, she couldn't comprehend how difficult it would be to have everything—even your recognizable gender—taken from you at such a vital age. Lexi decided to make headbands for these young women to wear as an alternative to hats. She took the time to create multiple headbands in various styles and colors to give these young women some options for accessorizing. She completed the project and met Cheryl at the cancer and hematology clinic to drop the headbands off. Little did she know that in only a few months' time, she would frequent that same clinic as a patient.

A month before Alexis's diagnosis, we had the opportunity to attend a star-raising party to celebrate Annika at the Make a Wish building. It was a festive occasion filled with treats, decorations, and Disney princesses. "This is so great!" Lexi said to Cheryl. "I love how excited the girls are and how much fun they are having. They are the cutest when they go sing and dance with the princesses."

"The princesses are actually a group of volunteers who volunteer for events like this, Lex. I can give you their information if you'd like it. You'd be amazing at it because of your personality," Cheryl replied.

"Are you serious?" Lexi said. "I'd love that! That would be so fun! I loved making the headbands, and I feel like I need to do something to be more involved."

"There is also a group of volunteers at the hospital called Kids Crew, who help out by playing with the kids who are inpatient or bringing them games and stuff. Some kids just do it because it looks good on college applications, but you'd be really great up there. You have to be fifteen, though. Didn't you just have your birthday?"

"Yeah, a couple of days ago. I'm so excited! That is so awesome! Do you have the information with you now?" Lexi asked. Cheryl quickly gave her the info and got back to the party.

As we were walking out to the car, we were once again talking about Lily, Annika, and the trials that cancer brings to a family.

"I just love them, Mom. They show me that no matter what happens in life, you can choose to be happy. Plus, I love how sassy Lily and Annika can be when they are singing and dancing." We both laughed as we did our best Lily and Annika moves.

"Mom," Lexi said as we got in the car, "you know how I've always wanted to be a cosmetologist when I grow up?"

"Yes."

"Well, I've been thinking that I need to do something that will help people. I need to be a nurse so that I can help more people."

"I think that's a wonderful idea, Lex. You have the perfect personality for that and have a way of putting people at ease. You'll be an amazing nurse. However, don't forget that a good cosmetologist has helped more people than you think!" We laughed and drove home talking about the plans she was making for her future.

As my mind recalled these memories and events just like them, I felt extremely blessed knowing that while nothing could fully prepare a family for cancer, we at least had the opportunity of being exposed to situations that made this transition much easier for our family. I watched in awe as the life we had seen others live, and that we openly commented on how we didn't know how they were able to do it, was now the life we would live. We were now classified as the strong, the brave, and the inspiring, though words such as "shattered," "broken," and "frail" would have been more suiting to the characteristics of my heart.

I found myself continually looking to Lexi to see how I could possibly shelter her from this storm. Never once did a shadow of a doubt cross her blue eyes. She refused to shrink in the face of a challenge. She knew the truthfulness of the words that had been spoken, and she would weather this storm with grace. Seeing her shoulders squared and her jaw set, I realized that she would overcome. She would rise. But it was more than a determination to survive. It was the knowledge that her life was exactly where it needed to be.

It became apparent early on that many people don't know how to react to cancer. It's like the club that everyone wants to admire from afar but nobody wants to join. The ugly face of cancer remains hidden from the majority of the world simply because it is too much for a person to voluntarily invest in emotionally. Even within the cancer community there are cancers that are more aggressive than others and thus drum up added sympathy from your cancer peers. A common coping mechanism is for parents or patients to discuss the treatment they have or will endure. It is a badge of courage that one is simultaneously proud of and loathes. Each patient and each family is suffering, and their suffering needs to be validated.

Before Lexi was diagnosed, I, along with much of the population, thought that cancer was difficult. I would look at a child with a beautiful bald head and think of how sad it was that they had to go through chemo and be sick. In my ignorance I did not fully understand the lengths to which the tentacles of this disease extend themselves. I knew that cancer ripped away many physical capabilities and attributes, but I was unprepared for the mental warfare that accompanied it. I was beginning to realize that my daughter would be challenged in ways she had never before been, and it would happen when she was at the weakest physical state of her young life. I would stand helplessly by and watch her be stripped down to the very core of who she was and pray that at the tender age of fifteen she would realize exactly what she was made of. She would experience things beyond what many could comprehend and what I could understand.

We had been at the hospital just less than a week when the day arrived for Lexi to get her port. This was the central line that all of her chemo and transfusions would go through, and it had a tube that led straight to my daughter's heart. This port would remain in place for several months. When it was not accessed (meaning there was no needle and line going into her skin), it looked like a small bump on her chest. It could be easily hidden and allowed her to shower and even swim without any precautions.

As odd as it sounds, there was a part of me that was grateful for her having a port. Logically it made sense. In the few days she had been there, Lexi had already been poked by IVs seventeen different times. It brought me comfort to know that she would now only be poked in one central location. However, comfort was not the only emotion that accompanied the placement of this port. Somehow this made cancer life more real. She really had cancer. They were really going to give her chemo. This was all real—our new reality.

Since diagnosis I had been updating people on Lexi's condition via Facebook. A friend had taken the liberty of setting up a group page for Lex, and before I knew it, people were flocking to it. Honestly, I couldn't understand why. Kids were being diagnosed every day, but somehow her story was spreading. She quickly became a recognizable face associated with childhood cancer—the tragic story of the teenage dancer with cancer. While the fact was that her condition was indeed tragic, we decided that our experience didn't have to be. I knew that if people were going to graciously follow us through this trial, I did not want it to drag them down. Rather, I wanted this experience to uplift them. I prayed that it would uplift me in the process.

My mind flooded with the trials that we had already overcome in this life and how we were able to overcome them. I was reminded that what got us through trials in the past was the same thing that would get us through our current situation. Several times, as things became cumbersome in my life, my dear bishop would remind me of the three most important priorities I would need to keep in order to be truly happy. If we were going to make it through this together, those same three things had to be our priority.

Our first priority was our individual relationships with God. Regardless of what had come or would come our way, we had to do everything we could to keep a strong relationship with Heavenly Father, not just as a family but also as individuals. He was the only one with the knowledge, power, insight, and complete perspective of our collective lives as a family, as well as our needs as individuals. My heart filled with gratitude as I realized that we had begun building our ark before this storm hit. Now we would need to do all within our power to preserve and protect this sacred relationship.

Our second priority had to be our marriage. Kris and I have been extremely blessed in our married lives. We've been through difficult challenges before but have always viewed them as us facing the world. Nothing has ever divided us. While cancer was no different in this area, we did find that the emotions we were experiencing were largely different. A father's primary role is to protect and provide for his family. Kris has always held his role as a father very sacred. He now found himself in a position where his daughter's life was in danger, and he could do absolutely nothing to protect her from the things she would have to endure to survive. As a mother, my primary role is to nurture and care for our children. While both of us would do anything to be able to take this pain from her, I was able to at least offset my grief by busying myself with things like helping her shower or holding her hand.

The root of the pain was the same; our responses to it were different. We were both hurting and helpless but for different reasons that needed to be expressed and understood by the other. For the first time in almost twenty years, we had to put concentrated effort into communication. "Kris and Emily" began before cancer, and if there was going to be "Kris and Emily" after cancer, there would need to be "Kris and Emily" during cancer.

Last, but no less important, our relationship with our kids had to be a priority. Like many parents, our children are our world. It was never our goal to be perfect parents. Is that really even a thing? Rather, our main objective has always been to make sure our children know that we love them and that they are a top priority in our lives. We knew they would not always agree with our parenting decisions, but we decided early on that our love for them would be the motivating factor in every decision we made. Now we were praying that as we had always loved them, they in turn would love and care for each other.

We talked openly and age appropriately with our children frequently, but even more important, we listened. We had a strong impression that their questions, concerns, and fears needed to be spoken aloud and addressed. There was no doubt that our situation was scary, but the unknown was frightening. Sometimes cancer and treatment was all they wanted to talk about, and sometimes they didn't want to even say the word "cancer" aloud. We talked about the things that would happen that we couldn't control. And more important, we talked about the things we could.

Chapter Five

When Tribulation Arises, Turn to the Lord

(Deuteronomy 4:30)

*I*t had been exactly one week from the day that I brought Lexi into the emergency room. It felt as if a lifetime had passed. She now had her port, and all of the necessary testing and the effects of chemo had been recited to us. Each day I watched as she became weaker and weaker—an effect of the ruptured tumor wreaking havoc on her insides. I marveled at the quick descent of the human body when it was under attack. Lexi was now considered a "falls risk," meaning she was unsteady on her feet, so we made sure that someone helped her each time she got out of bed.

It was the day of Lexi's first chemo, and because we didn't know how fast the nausea and fatigue would kick in, we opted to do her shower that morning instead of as part of her bedtime routine. She was sitting on the shower chair and said, "I haven't shaved my legs or armpits in over a week, Mom."

"Wow, Lex," I said jokingly, "that is disgusting."

She smiled, and a glimmer of sadness crossed her face. "Guess I won't really have to worry about that for much longer, huh?"

I nodded. "Well, why don't we just shave them today? I'll shave your legs and armpits and then braid your hair. You'll be looking fire for your first round of chemo!"

A smile played across her mouth. "You know, lots of people say that they have the best mom ever, but I really do. How many people can say that their mom shaved their legs and their armpits just so they'd look fire for chemo?" We laughed together, and I helped her dress and return to bed after her shower.

"You know, sis," I said once she was settled back in bed, "this change in your life means that we will be spending a lot more time together."

I'm not sure if it was the medicine kicking in or the high from the newly shaved legs, but her response warmed my heart nonetheless. "I know, and I'm so excited!" I wondered if there had ever lived a luckier mama.

The nurse walked in holding the poison that would save my child's life. She looked at the drugs that were scheduled to begin Lexi's treatment and said, "Oh wow! They're starting with these chemos?"

Being new to the cancer scene, I wasn't aware that there were some chemos that were harsher than others, but there are. Oftentimes a patient will receive a less harsh chemo to start with and then graduate to the harsher ones further in treatment. Apparently that wasn't an option for us. Again we were reminded that an aggressive cancer needed an aggressive treatment. Lexi would begin treatment by receiving cyclophosphamide (or cytoxan) and topotecan.

The plethora of accompanying side effects of many chemos are the same: extreme nausea, fatigue, loss of appetite, inability to heal from wounds or fight off infection, mouth sores, easy bruising or bleeding, and so on. In addition to this, cyclophosphamide is also known to burn the lining of the bladder, a condition known as cystitis. To offset this effect, an additional medication known as mesna is given in hopes of preventing this painful condition.

The act of receiving chemo is fairly anticlimactic in nature. The drugs are administered intravenously through a central line and then hung on a mobile IV pole or "tree" to allow the patient to be mobile if they are so inclined. Many children can walk around, play games, or watch movies while the chemo is being administered. To the unknowing onlooker, it may appear that the clear liquid entering the child's body is nothing more than a saline solution. The horrors that chemo holds are generally felt in the weeks, months, and years to come. It all depends on the patient and their body's response to the drug.

The biggest indicator that it is something more lies in the fact that the nurses administering the drugs have to wear shields and gloves to guard themselves from continued exposure. An internal struggle ensues when you see your nurse enter the room cloaked in protective gear to administer a drug through a tube leading directly to your child's heart that is so poisonous that they themselves need to take precautions. Lex rested in her bed as the medicine dripped into her body, sending a shiver down my spine and a pain through my chest. Our journey had officially begun.

During the delivery of chemo, our nurse asked me if we had seen the imaging of Lexi's tumor. I realized that with everything else that had happened, I hadn't even thought to look at the thing threatening my daughter's life since sleepily viewing it in the ER. At that time I was still focused on trying to find the elusive appendix so we could solve the problem and go home. She volunteered to pull up the imaging, and as she looked at it, she let out a low whistle. "This right here is why I am agnostic. If there is a God, why would He do this to a person like Lexi?"

I had never doubted the existence of Heavenly Father, and the past few days had reaffirmed my knowledge that He was there. However the question took me off guard. Was I really about to defend why my child had cancer? I silently prayed for understanding and direction. "I'm willing to open my mouth, Heavenly Father; I'm trusting you to fill it."

My mouth opened, and I realized that I was sharing a concept and simultaneously being taught that same concept. Throughout my life, I have heard people pose the question that if God really existed and He truly loved His children, then why would He allow them to suffer? The answer was actually simpler than I realized. Still uncertain of the words that would come out, I replied to the question posed by the nurse. "Do you have any children?" I asked.

"Yes . . ." she said, clearly unsure of where I was going with this. That made two of us. Nevertheless, I continued on.

"As parents we would do anything we could to keep our children from experiencing any unnecessary pain. However, when our kids were learning to walk, we had to let go of their hand from time to time and allow them to fall. It was the only way they would learn they had the strength to pick themselves up. Had we not, they would have never gained the ability to learn to walk on their own. They would not have realized the full potential of their capabilities had we taken that struggle from them. We had the power to spare them pain, but we also had the understanding that their struggle would ultimately benefit them. Instead of taking the obstacle from them, we stayed close by their side and helped them learn that they had the ability to overcome it."

I continued on. "I believe that the same concept applies as to why our Father in Heaven allows us to go through difficult challenges. Our limited perspective allows us to see only the immediate circumstances we find ourselves in. We focus on the hurt and the pain, rather than what is to be gained. If we, as imperfect as we are, hate to see our children suffer any unnecessary pain, how much more difficult is it for our Heavenly Father, in His perfect love and understanding, to see us struggle? Our suffering is something that He would allow only if He knew that it would ultimately be a blessing to us."

Our nurse looked at me as I smiled through tear-stained cheeks. Understanding had been given, but it didn't stop my heart from hurting at the knowledge of what my child would go through. I silently thanked my Heavenly Father for the newly acquired knowledge and the peace that somewhat eased the heartache. She nodded. "Huh . . . that actually makes sense." The topic changed back to cancer and the treatment ahead.

Once things had settled down and Lexi was resting in her bed, I took to the halls again. I ran into the lady who resided in the room next to ours—the fun room with all the decorations. Her name was Tracy, and her son Jake had been diagnosed earlier that year with AML (acute myeloid leukemia). They lived in Idaho but had been staying at the Ronald McDonald house in Salt Lake City during the course of Jake's treatment. During the past few months, the hospital had become their residence, because Jake had received a bone marrow transplant and his body needed to recover before leaving the hospital. Tracy's warm personality matched perfectly with the welcoming décor of their room. We talked openly, and I felt that I had made my first friend in this strange new world.

As we spoke just outside of her room, I saw the door open and a young boy appeared with a Red Sox baseball cap covering a completely bald head. He had more style than I did—his hat, shirt, shorts, and shoes were all color-coordinated. He smiled impishly as he inched his toes as close to the threshold of his room as he could get them and then wiggled the skin above his eyes (where his eyebrows should have been) as if to say, "Watch this!"

I watched as he playfully called out to his nurse. When he got her attention, he lifted one leg and swung it forward, crossing the invisible barrier from the room into the hall. "Jake," the nurse said in a mockingly stern voice, "you know you can't come out of that room yet."

"Technically I'm still in my room," Jake responded playfully. "Well, most of me is."

Amused that even cancer couldn't stop boys from being boys, I watched the exchange and turned to Tracy. "Why can't he leave his room?"

She responded, "When a child has a transplant or is neutropenic, meaning they have absolutely no immune system, they have to stay in their room to minimize exposure to any illness. Jake is allowed to come out once a day, usually around 10:00 p.m., to walk to the tub room. He has to bathe and go right back to his room. It has been that way for over a month now." I was speechless. This young man, so full of life, had been confined to a hospital room for over a month? How was Tracy still able to smile?

The answer came as she continued the conversation. "But this is the last step in his treatment. We are almost done! His counts are coming up, and from here we will just need to stay at the Ronald McDonald house for a few months, just to make sure he is doing well, and then we get to go home!" Her joy now made complete sense to me. While we were just beginning our journey, they were at the end of theirs.

"You guys should come out and watch Jake ring the bell," Tracy said.

"We'd love to," I replied. "But what exactly does that mean?"

She smiled. "They have a bell out by the nurse's station. The staff gathers around and they sing a little song, and the child who just completed treatment gets to ring the bell, signifying that they are done with their treatment. Do you guys want to come watch?"

"We wouldn't miss it!" I said, grateful for something to look forward to.

Two days later, we ventured out of our room, me pushing Lexi's wheelchair, and joined in the festivities of Jake's bell ringing. I stroked Lexi's hair as we sang, "No more, no more chemo . . . therapy" to the tune of "We Will Rock You." My heart swelled, and a tear ran down my cheek as I whispered to Lex, "That will be you one day, babe." She smiled and nodded. This act alone had officially solidified Jake as a hero in our hearts. He was the first kid we had ever seen firsthand who had beaten the monster we now faced. From that day forward, he became known by our family as "Jake who rang the bell," a title fit for a true warrior.

Chapter Six

She Had Faith No Longer, for She Knew

(Ether 3:19)

The days all seemed to run together, and before we knew it, it was September 23—Aleah's eighth birthday. We had hoped that Lexi would be finished with chemo in time to celebrate at home, but that just wasn't the case, so we improvised. Kris bought Aleah's presents and had Cam and Liv help wrap them. Then they all came up to the hospital, and we felt fortunate that Lexi was feeling well enough to leave her room. We celebrated with Del Taco (Aleah's favorite) in the Ronald McDonald room. This particular room is a large space that is patterned after a home. It has a kitchen area, where the food is communal and people are able to cook for themselves. It also has a computer area, a fireplace, and several chairs and couches where families can escape from the hospital room setting for a while.

We were lucky to spend some precious time outside the confinement of our hospital room, laughing, eating, laughing some more, and just enjoying each other's company while the last bit of chemo dripped into Lexi's veins. Her body seemed to already be sensing the attack, and she found that her appetite was being replaced by nausea and her energy by exhaustion.

Kris had taken the kids home, and I had taken Lexi back to the ICS floor to rest. "Tell me what you are thinking, Lex," I said as I glanced over to see her blue eyes gazing out the window of her hospital room. We had yet to make it home from the fateful ER trip.

"I feel as beat mentally as I am physically, Mama. Nothing gets a break. I'm worried about our family and stressed that I'm missing so much school. Chemo is insane. I knew it would be hard, but there aren't even words. Sick doesn't even begin to describe what it does to your body. I don't feel like me. I can't believe how weak I got, and it didn't even take long. I didn't know it was possible for someone to feel like this. It doesn't feel like any other sickness or weakness. It's completely different. I was blown away and so unprepared for this. I really don't know what could've prepared me for this."

The following day, the doctors came in to review with us the biopsy report that had been given by the surgeon. Again, I was in awe of the physical strength that Lexi's body had demonstrated. Her tumor had been largely displacing her pancreas and left kidney; it was pressing against her spine and encasing the arteries that supplied blood to many of her major organs. They asked how long prior to admission she had been unable to walk. I replied that she had gone to two practices and participated in three performances with her team the very day we came in. They simply looked at her and shook their heads. The strength and determination that her physical body had shown was inspiring, but the strength of her spirit was indescribable. They commented on her indomitable will. Lexi met the gazes of these learned individuals and humbly, yet matter-of-factly, stated, "I prayed before I performed that day. I asked Heavenly Father to help me do my best and to not let my team down. That is the only reason my body was able to do what it did."

I was astounded by her faith even more than I was by her physical strength. She had her moments of pain and sadness, but they were based on temporal things. She had no fear of whether or not she would be cured. None. It was more than faith; it was knowledge. She knew that if God said it through a priesthood blessing, it would come to pass. It was incomprehensible to me that a fifteen-year-old girl had this type of understanding, and yet she did. It was beyond words, and I was humbled to behold such a thing.

This faith was not something that was born overnight. It was gained line upon line and precept upon precept. When Lexi was seven years old, we told her that she needed to decide whether she would be baptized as a member of The Church of Jesus Christ of Latter-day Saints. As parents, we want the very best for our children. We want them to gain the knowledge and understanding that will help them become who they were intended to be. Kris and I had both experienced enough of life to know that a lasting happiness such as this was most likely to be obtained by following the principles of the gospel of Jesus Christ. It is not to say that happiness cannot be found in other ways, but this was what we knew to be best for our family. However, we knew that as much as we wanted that for our children, the decision ultimately needed to be theirs.

Eight sounds like a young age to make an everlasting covenant, but I've learned that at this very tender age, a child is still willing to learn, understand, and accept things that sometimes our stubbornness causes us to lose as adults. That being said, we prepared Lexi to make the decision to be baptized but reaffirmed that she had the final say in this process. It was a personal decision that needed to be taken seriously.

One night, after we had put Lexi to bed, she called me back into her room. I assumed this was an attempt to postpone bedtime, but the look in her eyes told a different story. She asked how she could know if God and Jesus were real, because she couldn't see them. I explained to her the importance of prayer, and if we honestly pray with our hearts, the Holy Ghost will help us know the truth of all things. I told her she needed to pray to find out for herself what was true. I left her room wondering if my message was beyond her young years.

Less than ten minutes later, she called me back in, her young eyes glistening. I asked if she was okay, and she responded, "Mom, Heavenly Father and Jesus are real. Satan is real too, and I want to get baptized right now."

Receiving a confirmation like that at such a young age imprinted on Lexi's soul the divine truths that she needed to know in order to fully trust Heavenly Father and His plan for her. Her faith continued to grow throughout her years. It was black and white. It was not just a belief; it was a knowledge. That knowledge helped her endure the unimaginable and look to the future without fear.

We had not yet resided in the cancer world for two weeks when we were told that Lex would need to be visited by a physical therapist. When a person is in the hospital for several days at a time, it is common for his or her muscles to deteriorate. Physical therapists come to assess each patient and his or her needs in order to try to prevent that from happening. Due to the pain from the tumor rupturing and the fact that she had started treatment, Lexi had been less than active lately. The physical therapist came into our room and asked if we could take a wheelchair ride down to the second floor where the therapy room was.

We arrived on the second floor, and the therapist asked Lexi to walk as far as she could while holding my hand so he could evaluate her strength. He knew her history and what she had been through over the course of the past week and was expecting Lex to stand from her wheelchair and walk a few yards before needing to sit down. He didn't understand the determination of our girl. She tightly held my hand and walked a full circle around the floor with the physical therapist asking her every few yards if she was ready to sit down. The longer she walked, the tighter her grip on my hand became. I could tell that the pain was taking its toll, but she was determined and focused. She refused to sit until she had completed the circle.

We used the wheelchair to get back upstairs. By the time she made it back to our room, she was shaking from the pain and the nausea. However, she didn't want to sit. She asked if she could try walking to the bathroom by herself. I let go of her hands but stayed near enough to catch her if her worn-out body gave out on her. I watched with tear-filled eyes as her feet slowly inched across the floor. I wanted nothing more than to reach out and stabilize her, but I knew she needed to do this on her own. Her fragile body slowly made it safely to its destination, and my heart rejoiced. Our daughter walked unassisted for the first time in almost two weeks. It was beautiful.

While Lexi was adjusting to what would be her new "norm" and preparing for life with cancer, Kris, Cam, Liv, and Aleah were making preparations of their own. We had plans to return home within the next day or so, and without us knowing, they had moved Lexi's bedroom from downstairs to upstairs to allow her easier access to the kitchen and the one bathroom in our home. Cam had willingly given up his room, which was considered prime real estate in our home, for a much smaller space. Together they had picked out a color, accessories, and took the time to paint their sister's new living area.

What many people do not realize is that when a child is given a diagnosis of such a serious illness, it not only changes their lives, but also the lives of each of their siblings—all in different ways.

Cam, being just barely thirteen, found himself needing to process emotions that he never knew existed. He had just learned that his best friend, the person he looked to for direction in every aspect of his life, was having her life threatened by something he couldn't even see. Cam and Lex had always held a very special bond. They shared the same due date and have an uncanny resemblance to one another, so their entire lives they have referred to one another as "twin." While most siblings love each other very much, the bond these two share is unique.

For the first time in his life, he struggled talking directly with Lexi, so his support came in other ways. He took a pen and wrote #AlexisStrong on his football jersey. He wore her bracelet every day and around his ankle in every football game he played. He found himself not only having to fill the role of the oldest sibling at home, but also that of caretaker while Lexi and I were in the hospital and Kris was at work. At perhaps one of the most pivotal times in his life, my young man's world came crashing down. He looked around helplessly, squared his shoulders, and did his best to begin rebuilding it.

Emotions are not generally something that teenage boys are completely comfortable talking about, and many times one emotion can manifest itself as another. Cam was a typical teenage boy in many aspects, but he had also been thrown an emotional curveball. It was now our job to distinguish between what was normal teenage boy behavior (is that even a thing?) and what had been caused by much deeper emotional frustrations. My mind was blank on the situation. However, I will never forget the lesson that we were able to learn so early on.

One afternoon, Cam had been asked to do something. He decided to exercise his agency and not do it. Consequences were enforced and frustration ensued. We were in his room trying to explain that while he can choose his actions, he cannot choose the consequences. He seemed to be getting so worked up over something so small. He was getting angrier, and I could tell that the situation was not nearing a resolution. I knew we were talking in circles, and I was exhausted. Just then, at the height of what I thought would be Cam's anger, Kris reached out and wrapped Cam, who was now almost his size, in the biggest dad hug I've ever seen. Immediately Cam broke down and began to sob uncontrollably. Kris just kept repeating, through a tear-filled voice, "It's going to be okay, Cam. Everything will be okay." I watched as father and son embraced and wept with one another. Nothing else needed to be said.

Upon hearing Lexi's diagnosis, Cameron's most prominent emotion was shock. Like all of us, he was surprised. We weren't a cancer family. We were an active family. A few weeks before diagnosis, we were camping and hiking together, and now his sister was stuck in a hospital room needing assistance to walk and breathe. It didn't add up. He had heard of people getting cancer and thought that it was so sad for them, but never would he have thought that we would be affected. Despite his concern, he said that he knew she would be okay. He said simply that the blessing she received right after diagnosis had given him the comfort that he needed to know that she would survive. That being said, he was not a fan of seeing any girl, let alone his big sister, suffer.

I felt myself get frustrated at the situation my family was in. Was it not enough that my child's life was being turned upside down, that one of my children was suffering? Now I was realizing that all of them were suffering. All of their lives were being turned upside down, and even after this event was over, nothing would ever go back to the way it was before. It was a hard pill to swallow.

Once again I felt helpless. The words I had spoken to my kids in a much different context came to my mind: "Don't focus on what you can't control; focus on the things that you *can* control." This event would have an immense impact on my children and their lives forever. As much as I wanted to, I couldn't control that their lives would be changed. However, we did have a say in how it would change. We could allow this experience to make us bitter, to fill us with anger and rage. Or we could allow this experience to make us better, to fill our hearts with love and understanding, with hope and faith. The choice was ours.

Chapter Seven

Our Hearts Were Full of Thanks
(Alma 37:37)

Almost as charming as the old storefronts of a small town are the traditions that the town carries. In Magna, one of the most illustrious traditions is known as "Blood Alley." Our local high-school mascot is the pirates, and the drill team that Lexi was a member of is known as the Cyprus Spinnakers. To honor graduating seniors in their respective clubs, distinguished members of the community, or homecoming royalty, the Spinnakers would form two lines and stand with their sabres drawn above their heads as the notable person walked beneath the outstretched blades. As the person passed by, the sabre was simultaneously twirled down and held at the side of each Spinnaker. It is one of Magna's most time-honored traditions and is reserved as a sign of honor.

We had just spent the last thirteen days in the hospital and found ourselves packing up with the knowledge that we would soon return. We loaded our belongings into our minivan and began the twenty-minute drive home, exhausted but grateful to be able to finally sleep under the same roof. We drove far enough that the four-lane highway eventually whittled down to just two lanes, and then we exited. The llamas grazed in the open space just off the highway exit, and we passed the same old store that had gone from flower shop, to themed gift shop, to car dealership, all within the past ten years.

We took the next turn to our home, and my eyes caught sight of large purple ribbons that had been tied to every pole we passed. A friend had sent us a picture of her handiwork and told us that the purple was to signify neuroblastoma awareness on Lexi's behalf. Although I had looked at the picture several times, it did not do it justice. Something about experiencing the love and support first hand, something about seeing this very visible evidence of awareness from the community we so dearly loved, made my heart swell. Everything was the same as it had always been, and yet somehow everything had changed.

We pulled into our neighborhood, and my heart quickened. We were so close to being home again together that I could feel it in my bones. As we neared our home, we saw a few extra cars, and lining our driveway were numerous Spinnakers still in their practice clothes, standing at attention. We pulled our white minivan, complete with the newly affixed #AlexisStrong decal spreading across the rear window, up to the curb.

We opened the door to the sound of the drill president saying, "Salute sabre!" Tears fell down my face as Lexi's Spinnie sisters stood at attention on either side of our driveway. Still feeble from the treatment, Kris came to her aid as Lexi gingerly exited the car. Slowly she walked through Blood Alley supported by Kris on one side, me on the other, and her team lifting her spirit. Girl after girl held her sabre high with tears in her eyes as Lexi passed. At the end of Blood Alley stood Cam with Liv and Leah holding a sign welcoming their sister home. She made it to the end, and we all embraced. The Spinnies broke ranks and joined the embrace with tear-stained faces.

While in the hospital, we were oblivious to many of the goings-on in our community. We would see the occasional picture or receive a message about things that were happening, but our minds had been so focused on comprehending this new life that we didn't have strength for anything else. However, we were told about a football game happening at Lexi's high school that Friday night. We had cleared it with her doctors and got the okay to go. Our friends had brought us shirts sporting the signature #AlexisStrong logo. Our whole family put on our shirts and went to the game together.

We entered the local football stadium as we had so many times before, only this time Lexi would watch the game from a wheelchair instead of the bleachers. There would be no sequined costume or glitter makeup tonight. As we entered the old, familiar stadium, we heard the announcer's voice tell the story of a beautiful fifteen-year-old girl who had tragically been diagnosed with cancer. My initial thought was, "How sad for that sweet girl. That would be so difficult!" My head then had to remind my heart that the sweet girl they were talking about was *my* sweet girl.

We made our way to the home side of the field, and the principal had special seating for us on the track to minimize the direct contact Lexi would have with people, in hopes of avoiding illness. Despite the barrier, several people approached her, offering their well wishes, condolences, and support. Lexi is not one who requires a spotlight to shine. In fact, in many cases she tries to avoid it, but there would be no avoiding it on this night. We didn't mind though. It did our hearts good to once again be surrounded by the people we loved so dearly. The first half of the game was coming to an end, and we were escorted as a family to the fifty-yard line for the halftime presentation. While we waited for the final seconds to tick off of the clock, I noticed that at the back of each boy's helmet a yellow sticker had been placed. It read simply #AlexisStrong.

The referees whistled, indicating that the first half had come to an end. We continued the walk to our designated halftime seats. We passed by the cheerleaders, who in unison sang the words my heart had been screaming for the past two weeks: "Fight, Lexi, Fight!"

The crowd, many of whom were wearing shirts with Lexi's name on them, joined the battalion with the chant of "We are . . . Alexis strong!" Hundreds of people in our small community were joining their voices with those around them to show their support for our family in this, our greatest moment of weakness.

We sat huddled together at the center field sideline as we watched Lexi's drill team take the field for the first time without her. My heart stopped as they walked out. Each of the girls was holding hands with the girl next to her—united. Their shirts read, "I aspire to be Alexis Strong." Tears welled up in my eyes, and I let them spill over. Honestly, after the past two weeks, I was in awe that I actually had any tears left to shed, but apparently they replenish quite quickly.

A lump formed in my throat as the music began. For the next two minutes, my eyes were fixed on twenty-five girls, not twenty-six, who were dancing to words of hope and courage, words of strength and fight, words of love. They had choreographed and learned a dance in a few short days to show Lexi their support in an unspoken language that they all shared. The dance concluded, and everyone was on their feet. Optimism, sadness, and heartache lobbied to be the prominent emotion of the night, but unity conquered them all.

The announcer then said that they would be holding a "miracle minute" for our family. He encouraged those present to donate what they could to the student body officers, who would be coming around the stands. Any funds donated would go directly to helping offset the cost that our upcoming battle would hold. We were amazed to learn that in just one minute's time our family and friends raised over $2,000. In a community where people live paycheck to paycheck, we were literally receiving the widow's mite.

We were told that another announcement was to be made, and our family was escorted to the center of the new turf field. There we were met by a good friend of ours, who told us that an anonymous donor had donated $40,000 to Primary Children's on our behalf. My heart stopped. I looked to Kris, who just grabbed me, Lex, Cam, Liv, and Leah. We embraced there on the pirate logo in the middle of the field, collectively sobbing at what we had just learned. As he pulled back, Kris's blue eyes held a sense of complete relief as he felt the financial burden of this trial lifted from his shoulders.

We knew Lexi's treatment would be expensive. We knew it would strain our already tight budget, but that had not been our concern. Our only thought was that we would do whatever needed to be done in order to assure that our daughter got the best physical care possible. There would be nothing she needed that we wouldn't provide, even if doing so cost all of our worldly possessions. In this one moment, we learned that it wouldn't have to. This one donation caused the entire financial burden up to this point to be negated. My heart swelled as I felt such gratitude for this faceless stranger with such a giving heart.

We walked back to our seats as the game commenced. A woman we did not personally know approached Lexi and handed her a folded up two-dollar bill. "This has been carried in my wallet for over a decade. It has brought me good luck, and now I want to pass it on in hopes that it will do the same for you." Lexi thanked her graciously, touched by the personal gesture, and they embraced. That same bill has been carried in my wallet ever since that night.

Some of the local news channels had been informed of the night's event and had come out to our little community to cover the proceedings. After the halftime presentation, a few of the reporters asked us to expound on our feelings regarding the large donation. As I thought about it, I realized that while we were sincerely grateful for the donation that would cover many costs of Lexi's treatment, to us it held no higher place than that of the two-dollar bill that had been given to Lex. What was truly amazing to us had nothing to do with the amounts of money that had been donated but the love with which it was given.

"People from outside of our community may be surprised by the generosity that was shown here tonight," I told the reporter, "but I am not. We are blessed to live among people who truly care and want to help one another in whatever way they can. We are more than a community. We are a family. This event was just evidence of what we already knew." We spent the rest of the night together visiting with friends and family while cheering on our high school football team.

I've heard about the roller coaster of emotions that accompany the cancer life, but I was not ready for how soon we would experience the ride. It was now late Saturday night, just twenty-four hours after the big football game. We had been home from the hospital for a measly two days, and Lexi was running a fever. At this point I had been a mom for over fifteen years and had learned that fevers are just the body's way of fighting off an infection. However, in a child with no immune system, a fever can prove to be deadly and requires immediate hospitalization.

So again we found ourselves in the hospital. We had gone from seeing and feeling the strength and love of our friends, family, and community to once again being isolated in our small room. Lexi was hooked up to an IV so she could receive antibiotics while they monitored her and waited for her fever to break. We were extremely lucky that time—we were only there an additional three days.

Somehow we had made it through the last two and a half weeks. We were home together and were trying to establish new routines that coordinated with our new life. We found ourselves needing to reside in two different worlds—a world where school, practices, and regular bedtimes ensue, and a world where there are no guarantees, all plans are fluid, and children literally fight for their lives every day.

Lexi was still on oxygen (she had yet to be taken off of it since diagnosis), and her body was extremely weak from the beating that the chemo had delivered. But she had pictures with her drill team the following day and needed a new outfit. The last time I had been shopping with Lexi was a few days before I took her into the emergency room. We had spent the afternoon looking for a homecoming dress, and after hours of giggling and trying on dress after dress, we were heading home with just a great pair of red heels. It had been a careless afternoon of laughter and silliness. This experience was nothing like that.

I headed to Target like I had countless times, looking for a black outfit for Lexi's team pictures just like we did a year ago. But this time I had to take into account that Lexi wasn't with me. It wasn't because she was at practice or out with her friends. She wasn't with me because she didn't have the strength to go shopping with me like she had done a hundred times before. She wasn't with me because we didn't know how busy the store would be and didn't want to risk her getting sick and running another fever. She wasn't with me because she had cancer.

In addition to that, I realized that this outfit—the first outfit I would buy her since she was diagnosed—had to account for her weight loss and needed to cover her port. Everything about this felt wrong. It seemed as if every mother-daughter duo in the tristate area was at that particular Target at that particular moment, yet I found myself alone.

My ears caught bits and pieces of conversations as I meandered about the store aimlessly. I overheard someone talking about what a bad day they'd had. Their bad day consisted of the milk being gone in the morning, their hair not curling in the right direction, and traffic on their way to work. My mind raced. I remembered those bad days. I longed for them.

But I could not compare my life to someone else's if I was to find happiness. My trials were difficult, but they were mine. I was built to handle them, even when I didn't feel like I could.

"Adam fell that men might be; and men are, that they might have joy" (2 Nephi 2:25). We were created to be happy, to enjoy life, and that would not happen if we were focusing on the negative aspects of this or any trial. In order to be happy, we would have to actively pursue every good thing in our lives. We could no longer wait for happiness to come; we would have to seek it out. With a new perspective and a new resolve, I finished the task at hand so I could return home to my family, grateful for the opportunity to do so.

The next day, as I drove Lexi to her team pictures, we tried to make small talk. She had taken special care how to wear her dark brown hair that day—both of us knowing this would likely be the last professional picture she would have taken before it all fell out. She opted to wear it loosely curled and cascading over her shoulders and down her back. Drill team pictures are always taken on location, and this year they had decided to take the pictures in downtown Salt Lake City. Lexi's body was still very weak from her treatment. So, instead of a makeup bag and the usual accessories for pictures, we brought along enough medication to see a small village through a crisis, multiple masks (although we were going to be outside we didn't know what the air quality would be like), a wheelchair, and an oxygen tank. I had first parent syndrome all over again.

Kris met us downtown and opted to stay with Lex just in case she got too tired, too sick, or there was a zombie apocalypse. We were prepared for it all. I parked, and together we unloaded her unlikely accessories. He spent the following few hours pushing her wheelchair to various locations and carrying her on his back to the locations that the wheelchair could not go. She was able to take her oxygen off occasionally and smile for various pictures. In addition to team pictures and head shots, each girl did an action shot to showcase their strongest dance ability. Action shots are often thought of well before picture day and are usually the favorite pose since it highlights a young woman's beauty as well as her talent.

It came time for Lexi's action shot to be taken. Kris carried her up some stairs on his back and set her down. Her oxygen had been left behind for a moment. She used an old tree branch to steady herself behind a thin waterfall. She held tightly to the tree branch with one hand and with the other she grabbed her right ankle. She took a breath and raised her leg up to her head and then tilted toward the branch.

A few months later we got the proofs of these pictures. I opened them up and was speechless. I remember that day as the day we unloaded her baggage and a piece of my heart. I remember it as the day she was no longer free to run from place to place with her friends, the day I dropped her off for pictures and then cried by myself the whole way home. But her pictures told a different story. I did not see a young woman who was beginning the fight of her life, or a child who had tragically been diagnosed with cancer. I saw only my daughter doing what she loved.

A few days after her team pictures, we were able to attend Cam's football game together, just like we always did. Kris had coached Cam every year that he had played, and that year was no different. When Lexi was diagnosed, many people asked Kris why he continued to coach. "There are more important things than football to worry about," they would say.

"Yes," he responded, "there are more important things than football, but nothing is more important than our children. This is my time with my son. It always has been, and we both need it now more than ever." Needless to say, Saturday morning football continued to be a staple in our schedule.

We pulled up to the field and began the trek to the game. Lex was still in her wheelchair, so making it to the sideline came with a little more effort than normal. We did our best to navigate her wheelchair as smoothly over the uneven grass as possible. I could see her grasping the arm holds with each bump. Liv and Leah stayed faithfully by our side as we continued the struggle. A friend saw our predicament and came over to offer assistance, another friend following closely behind him. They lifted the chair and carried Lexi across the grass as I held Livi's and Aleah's hands tightly in mine. We thanked our dear friends for their help and silently thanked Heavenly Father for sending them. We neared the neatly laid out fields like we had so many times over the years. However, this time something was different.

As we approached the field, I realized that something had been painted in the end zone. Upon further examination, I recognized that every end zone had been carefully spray painted with the words #AlexisStrong. My heart swelled within me, and I could feel the water rising in my eyes once again. I didn't even try to stop it anymore. This was not done for Lex—we didn't even know if she would be able to come to this game today. This had been done for Cam, for Kris. It was a way to show them that their football family was right beside them in this fight.

As we neared even closer, my heart leapt again as I saw a sticker attached to the back of each helmet in the shape of a purple ribbon accompanied by the words #AlexisStrong. We were truly a team. The boys played that season with more heart than I had ever seen. They played for Kris, for Cam, for Lex, for each of us. They lost only to the state champions. They will forever be our boys.

Chapter Eight

The Very Hairs of Your Head Are Numbered

(Matthew 10:30)

*O*ne of the most recognizable effects of chemo is hair loss. For some patients it is a thinning of hair, and for others it is complete and total baldness. We were told upon starting treatment that Lex would be bald for at least one year and that she could begin losing her hair within one to two weeks of receiving her first dose of chemo. Right then and there I made a decision. "Lex, I'm going to shave my head," I told her. When your child is going through something like this, there are so many things that you cannot experience with them. This was something I could do, something I wouldn't just have to sit by and idly watch as she endured it on her own.

She looked at my long, dark hair. "Mama, you have great hair. I don't want you to cut it."

"It's just hair," I responded. "Plus, I don't want it. I've been looking for a reason to change things up, and now I have that reason. You can do it if you want. We will make a party out of it!"

Somehow it felt like a betrayal for me to keep my hair when she couldn't keep hers. Why should I have hair when my child could not? I begged her to let me do this, to let me cut my hair, but she begged me not to. I let the conversation drop, but my mind would not let it go.

I thought to myself, "This is how I can support her. This is something I can do. She probably doesn't know how much of a support it would be or how good she will feel seeing the physical evidence of her not being alone in this journey." Days passed, but she didn't budge on the topic. I tried to approach it from every angle and got nowhere. I knew that ultimately it was my hair and my decision, but what was my motivation? Was this really for Lexi?

I meekly admitted that in trying to offer a support or service, I was focusing on my needs, not hers. If I were to shave my head, it would be only to make me feel better; as if there was something I could do in a situation where I felt utterly helpless.

There are many people who would feel uplifted and supported if those closest to them shaved their heads to embrace the bald life together. I wanted to be that support. I've heard stories of dads who let their child with cancer shave their head to lessen the fear of having a bald head, or husbands who shave their heads in support of their wives, groups of friends who make a party of going bald together. However, that was not Lexi. She wouldn't want anyone to go through anything unnecessarily—especially on her behalf. If I went through with it, instead of looking at me and seeing support, Lexi would look at me and be reminded of how everything in her life had drastically changed, even my appearance. If I went through with this, it would be for me, not her.

My heart ached as I realized that the one thing I felt I could do was not what she needed. She didn't need me to physically show my support to her and the rest of the world. She needed me to quietly hold her hand while she slept, cradle her when she cried, and scream for her when she couldn't. If I was going to be a strength to her, I would need to put aside all of my own feelings about what was emotionally best for her and rely solely on what she told me and the inspirations that Heavenly Father would give me.

This was without a doubt the most painful thing I've ever gone through, but this trial was not about me. This trial was about my child, and I prayed to find my role in it. My body has never physically experienced cancer the way that hers would. I could not tell her what to expect or how it would feel. My knowledge of what she needed was so very limited—but Heavenly Father knew.

My prayers changed and focused not only on her needs but also on the needs of Kris, Cameron, Olivia, and Aleah as well. I had been a wife for seventeen years and a mother for fifteen, and suddenly I was at a loss as to what would be best for my family. I had to rely completely on the mercies of Heavenly Father to help me understand how I could best be of service to each of them. Above all, pride in any form had to be abandoned, and love had to continue to be the motivating factor for my actions.

I thought of Lexi's long, thick brown hair and had hope that she might not lose all of it. Maybe with some creative styling she could just change things up a bit and no one would be the wiser. How wrong I was. She had made it through the first chemo treatment, and now we waited to see just how quickly and harshly the effects of these drugs would begin to assault her. It began only eight days after her first treatment had concluded. She ran her fingers through her hair and found that her hands contained several strands of her precious locks. It had begun.

Losing your hair is not physically painful. The cells die, and the hair falls out several strands at a time. "Do you want to try some wild new haircut or dye it some insane color before it all falls out, Lex?" we asked, trying to lessen the heaviness of what she must be feeling.

She wistfully smiled and replied, "No, it's okay. I just want to keep my hair long as long as I can. I know it's just hair and it doesn't really matter, but it just makes everything so real. I really have cancer. I'm really going to be bald. It's all real." Over the next several days, a routine was developed in our home.

Multiple times a day I sat behind Lexi with a brush. Because of how long her hair was, it quickly matted as it fell out. Olivia, Aleah, and Kris took turns alternating between hand holders. This very important position also required one to wipe away the few tears that managed to escape Lexi's clear eyes. Whoever was not on hand-holding duty would take the large balls of hair directly from my hand to the garbage. When the brushing was complete and what was left of her hair was unmatted, Cam would immediately take the garbage outside so that his sister did not have a visual reminder of the impending effect of her treatment. It took only a few short days for her hair to be almost completely gone.

The day had come that Lexi felt comfortable shaving off the final strands of her beautiful locks. I had placed what was left of her hair into a very small braid at the base of her neck. A close friend that Lexi loved dearly was kind enough to agree to shave Lexi's head at her in-home salon. This offered a more intimate setting for a very personal moment. Kris, Lex, and I arrived at Jessica's home and walked down to the salon entrance. She greeted Lex with a warm hug and motioned for her to sit in the barber chair. "Should we give you a mullet or a mohawk?" Jessica said, trying to lighten the mood.

Lexi smiled and shook her head. "Let's just get rid of it."

Jess then asked Lex if she wanted to do the honors of cutting off her miniscule braid. With a twinkle in her eyes, Lexi looked at me. "Mom, you do it. You said it was on your bucket list to cut off a rat tail—here is your chance!" I mustered up a giggle that she had even thought of that and assured her that this was not the same thing, but she was insistent. Lexi is nothing if not determined when she has made up her mind, so I reluctantly agreed.

I held the scissors and forced a smile. If she needed this to be a silly experience, I was not going to stop her. I held my breath and cut off the last of my daughter's hair. I then took one of her hands in mine and Kris took the other in his. Together we watched helplessly as, once again, our daughter tightened her jaw and accepted the trial she had been given. My heart shattered as I watched a single tear run down her cheek. Her eyes were distant, and any laughter was long gone. The room was silent except for the sound of the clippers, which seemed to scream that life was not fair.

The entire process took but a few short minutes to complete. I looked at Lexi again to see that more than just her appearance had changed. Her countenance had changed also. We have been blessed with beautiful daughters, but we wanted them to grow up know-ing that true beauty is based on character, not physical attributes.

When Lexi's hair, one of her beautiful physical attributes, was gone, it revealed a beauty that I had previously not seen. She was stunning. She literally radiated beauty. I was speechless. I had always told her how beautiful she was, and I even expected her to look cute with a bald head, but I wasn't prepared for this. Her smile was more welcoming, the light sprinkling of freckles across her nose was more prominent, and her eyes shone more brightly. I knew she had accepted this life, but until this moment, I didn't recognize that she would embrace it.

A company had generously offered to donate a beautiful, real human hair wig to Lexi in exchange for a few photos of her wearing it. I had talked to her previously, and she said she was comfortable with that. So, upon having her head shaved, and when she felt ready, the representatives from the company entered the room with the wig. She tried it on, talked about it, and did a few photos. However, when she got into the car, I asked her if it was something she would be wearing regularly. She replied, "I don't think so. It is normal for kids with cancer to be bald. There is nothing wrong with it." I wholeheartedly agreed, and from that time on, hats were worn only to keep her naked head warm or protect it from the sun. The remainder of the time was spent showcasing that bald is, in fact, beautiful.

Chapter Nine

Her Mouth Shall Speak Truth

(Proverbs 8:7)

*T*he weeks in between our next round of chemo were spent enjoying—truly enjoying—our time together. We now appreciated the company of one another in a way that we had never before. We got to laugh and play games and have movie night. I got to help my kids get ready for school and drive their carpool. I got to kiss Kris and tell him to his face that I loved him every single day. It is not that anything drastic had changed in our regular routines—these are things that we had always done. Rather it was our perspective of how truly blessed we were to be able to do them.

There is no vacation from fighting cancer—trust me; I checked into it. If a patient is not being poked and prodded in the hospital, he or she is being poked and prodded at home. The extent of home care depends largely on a patient and his or her particular treatment plan. For us, we learned quite early to become proficient in IV antibiotics and medications, TPN (IV nutrition), fluids, feeding tubes, and injections. However, we were still not qualified for our biweekly blood draws and nurse check-ups. For that, we were lucky enough to have Nurse Cheryl. Cheryl was the first nurse to come into our newly diagnosed cancer home. Her soft demeanor and sincere concern coupled with her clear knowledge of all things medical quickly won the hearts of our family. Although I was sure that there were many other patients she had to see, she had a way of making Lexi feel like she was her favorite. I'm certain that all of her patients would say the same thing. A relationship quickly developed, and we found ourselves looking forward to our visits from Nurse Cheryl as a visit from a friend.

The time came for us to go back to the hospital for Lexi's second round of chemotherapy. We were hopeful that this time we would be staying in the hospital for only a week. During this visit, we had a CT scan that showed that the tumor was slightly smaller than it was when we started. We figured that even the smallest of victories should be celebrated, but this one came with a caveat. The CT also found some spots on Lexi's liver that had previously not been detected. Discussions were had by her team of doctors, and the conclusion was reached that whether these spots were cancerous or not, her treatment would remain the same. We would stay the course and continue to pray that no more surprises lay in store.

While the results of the CT did not affect her treatment plan, recent studies that had been completed did. A doctor from the bone marrow team came into our humble hospital room as the second round commenced. He sat on a stool at the end of Lexi's bed and told us that he had just returned from a medical conference. New data had been released that showed that if a patient with neuroblastoma underwent two stem cell transplants as opposed to one, the likelihood of relapse fell from 55 percent to 45 percent. These odds were still not great, but at least now they were on our side of the coin. While I tried to be optimistic, the words from a conversation that I'd had earlier with Tracy, Jake's mom, were instantly brought back to my mind.

"They said Lexi will need a transplant. Is it really as bad as I've heard?" I asked, hoping that my concerns were irrational.

"It's worse," she replied matter-of-factly. "The chemo they give your child right before transplant is fatal if the transplant doesn't take. Your child becomes a bag of organs while they fight to stay alive."

I exhaled and brought myself back to the present. I told myself that I could revisit this conversation on a sleepless night, for today

I had to focus on the fact that the odds were flirting with the idea of being in our favor. This study had been taking place over the past twenty years and had just now been released and approved as standard care. For once, it seemed like the timing of this cancer was somewhat of a blessing, and right now I needed to focus on recognizing the blessings in my life in whatever form they manifested.

Lexi's treatment plan, or road map, as they called it, would now consist of three more rounds of chemo, followed by surgery to remove the tumor. A sixth round of chemo would be next. She would then endure two stem cell transplants. After the transplants, she would undergo radiation and then six rounds of antibody therapy. At this point, she would be evaluated again to see what our next step was. Still, they offered no false hope of an end in sight.

I stepped out of the room to call Kris at work and update him on the new findings and added treatment. As expected, he was not thrilled with the idea of Lexi having another transplant. However, we all had the end goal in sight—to get Lexi cancer free—and we would all do whatever was necessary to reach that goal. He then told me that he had spoken to our friend who had acted as the liaison between Kris and I and the anonymous donor at the football game. "It turns out that over the past week the donor has been avoiding phone calls. They've followed up with Primary's, and nothing has been donated. They were able to find out who the donor is, and he doesn't have the money. There is no donation."

"Do you know who it is?" I asked.

"Yes," he responded, "but we know his child better." Kris told me the name of the donor, and I instantly knew that there was no way the donation would happen. It wasn't that the act was malicious. I'd like to believe that the person involved simply didn't have the means to make it happen. Oddly enough, we both still felt at peace. Yes, we had just learned that perhaps we were not as financially prepared for this battle as we thought we were a week ago, but that didn't change the fact that our end goal was still the same. We would do whatever was necessary to make sure that Lexi was cancer free.

Word travels fast in a small town, and when you are more like family than friends, people become protective—especially in time of crisis. We knew that this development would spread like wildfire, so we did our best to stop the fire from starting. Our friend who acted as the liaison contacted the news stations that covered the story and asked them to print a retraction. From our standpoint, we posted an update on all of our social media pages in hopes of minimizing the impact that this revelation would have on the members of the family of the false donor. We asked that the person's name be left out of any mention of the event, as he had children in the community. We did not want any backlash on the child from his peers. A child is worth far more than $40,000. Magna is a small community, and we knew that word would travel. So we asked that our friends and members of our community do all that they could to minimize the effect that this event could potentially have.

Despite the setback, we didn't feel anger or hate. Like I said before, those were emotions that we just didn't have the strength to hold onto. But it was more than just lack of energy that caused the would-be frustration to subside. It was that we were trying to keep our focus on the things that mattered, and in doing so, our under- standing of what was truly important had been made clear. By not allowing our focus to stay on the negative event, our minds were free to recognize the blessings we had been given. We felt a genuine love and appreciation for those around us and for the care and concern they continued to show our family during this difficult time.

We felt blessed that the false donation and the surrounding chaos was the only major bump during our second round of chemo. We were able to return home in just a week's time, and that was never something to be taken lightly. We would enjoy three weeks together before needing to return for round three. However, that didn't mean we got three weeks completely free. We would still need to return to clinic at least weekly for labs, transfusions, and general check-ups, and more often if she showed any of the "worry signs" they had told us to watch for. But those were all minor setbacks. Ultimately, life was good, and we were learning to be truly grateful for the things that mattered.

During treatment, a patient needs to consistently be monitored for multiple things. Much of this monitoring can be done outpatient to minimize hospital stays. Blood draws or labs are a regular occurrence and can be performed at home or in clinic. This requires blood to be drawn and then tested for things such as red and white blood cell counts (indicating function of blood cells, infection, or lack of immune system), platelet counts, and kidney and liver function, just to name a few. This is a regular occurrence to screen whether a child is healthy enough to proceed with the next round of treatment, if he or she needs a transfusion, or if the child's body just needs more time to try to recover on its own. Certain chemo can also be done in clinic. The child can come and get his or her infusion and return home. Some children are able to get much of their treatment outpatient because of the services that the clinic offers.

Upon walking into the clinic, you are greeted by a lovely receptionist with a welcoming smile. You sign the name of the patient and then wait in the small waiting room until the patient is called. Once called, the patient is taken to a chair that is next to a long desk. The patient's weight and vitals are taken and recorded on their chart. When this is done, the patient is told he or she can sit back in the waiting room if the patient is healthy enough to do so. If not (due to a contagious illness or if he or she is a transplant patient), the patient is then escorted to his or her own private room.

If a patient is healthy and is there only for a transfusion or an outpatient chemo, he or she is taken to the back of the clinic, which resembles a busy InstaCare. A recliner for the patient is set next to a rocking chair for whoever is accompanying them. Privacy can be attained by pulling a curtain closed around the miniscule area. Snacks are provided if a patient feels up to eating, and games abound if they have enough energy to play.

On this particular Monday, we had come to the clinic only to get labs drawn. As we entered, I looked around and recognized this as the exact place we had brought the headbands just a few months before. I smiled sadly at the irony. We had been home for a full week and were planning on spending the next two weeks sleeping in our own beds. We were taken to a room and were awaiting lab results to see if our hour-long lab appointment would turn into a four-hour-long visit because she needed a transfusion. Cancer teaches you early to prepare for the worst but hope for the best.

Lexi's labs came back, and the doctors came in looking surprised and pleased. This demeanor was easily picked up on, because it was rarely seen in our room. They said that Lexi was actually healthy enough to do the stem cell collection that day. Her body had been reacting well to the shots that she had been getting at home and was a little ahead of what they had planned. We were told that she could be admitted right then. A central line catheter would be placed in her neck and then over the course of the next day or two, her stem cells would be collected to be used for her transplants later in treatment.

We called Kris, and together we decided that there was no time like the present. This would have to be done at some point, and we were anxious to cross off any steps on our road map as quickly as we could. It made it feel like we were making progress instead of just standing still. Kris came to the hospital with a few provisions we would need for our short stay. He stayed with me as, again, they listed the possible side effects of anesthetic and why the line needed to be placed.

A small procedure was done in which a large catheter, or tube, was placed into Lexi's jugular vein. This is a vein in the neck where there is a large amount of blood flow, making the collection easier. Just over an hour passed when we were called and told that Lexi was done and ready for us. We met her in the recovery room and immediately took note of the straw-sized tube protruding out of our daughter's neck.

The combination of Lex and anesthetic was one that no one wanted to miss out on. Despite the new hardware, she was as chatty as ever. I quickly learned that the fears I carried while she was under anesthetic dissipated as soon as I could hear her rambling. The mood was instantly lightened by us asking random questions and listening to her candid responses. It was a good thing that she had always been such an open and honest person, because I'm not sure that she had the ability to keep a secret when she was coming off of anesthetic, even if she'd tried.

"So, Lex," I said, winking at the nurses and nodding a little, "tell me what you think about this particular boy." I would give her the name of different young men, and she would reply with a completely uncensored opinion of that young man.

She was even quick to clarify between "friend-friends" and "cute-friends." If there was a moment that wasn't filled with talking, Lexi began rambling about anything and everything, so I continued to ask her questions in hopes of steering the conversation away from things I figured she probably didn't want the entire free world to know. The time came that Lexi was stable enough to head back to our room.

"Okay babe, we are going to start going back to the room. The nurses will push your bed, and dad and I will be right beside you."

"Wait, Mom," she said. "Why do we have to go so soon? I'm having fun right here."

"Well, they have other patients coming, and they need the room for those patients."

"Who's coming?" she said.

"I don't know their names, sweetheart. They can't tell us their names because of patient confidentiality," I replied.

"But I just want to be their friend. I'm trying to make friends, Mom. How can we be friends if I don't know their name 'cause of confidentiality?"

A tech then came to my aid. "Lexi," she said, "I thought we were friends! Can I be your friend?"

Lexi looked right at her, grinned from ear to ear, and held up her pointer finger. "You are my *best* friend!" The nurses all laughed as Lex continued on about her new bestie. Knowing she had made a new friend kept Lexi content enough that we could leave the recovery room.

The laughter continued as they escorted us back to our room. "I'm so tired of talking, Mom," Lex said as the elevator took us back to the fourth floor, "but I just can't stop." I stifled a laugh, and it occurred to me that laughter and joy could be and should be found in any setting.

We were just getting situated when I looked at her and said, "Man, we are a good time, Lex!"

She got a big smile on her face and replied, "Yeah, we are. Our family is always a good time. Nothing—not even a little cancer—is going to stop us from having fun." I'm not sure that the doctors would agree that high-risk neuroblastoma was just "a little cancer," but I had to admire her optimism.

We got completely settled back in our room and were waiting for the collections technician to come in and begin the process of collecting the stem cells. "Do you care if I take a picture, Lex?" I asked while we were waiting. "With your bald head and those lines sticking out of your neck, you kind of look like a babe of a robot." Her eyes flashed a hint of edginess, and she instantly formed a peace sign, accompanied with a sassy pair of duck lips. I laughed out loud and snapped a photo.

The technician entered our room and explained the collection process in a little more detail. The catheter would be hooked up to a machine that resembled the machines used to collect plasma—only this one was much louder and more obnoxious. The machine would extract her blood and spin it, keeping the plasma and stem cells, and then return the rest of her blood to her body. While the collection was taking place, the technician was not allowed to leave our room, so for the better part of two days we had a stranger set up shop in our already-crowded hospital room. It was a different technician each day, and although they were nice enough, we were grateful to have a small sense of privacy when the collection was complete.

Over the course of two days, they were able to collect enough stem cells for three transplants. The doctors said that they had two transplants planned and enough cells "for a rainy day." I was grateful for their foresight but felt we had already had enough rain. I was ready for a rainbow. "If Lexi ends up not needing it and you are okay with it, the cells will go on to help another patient or be used for research purposes." I wholeheartedly agreed, hoping that someone, somewhere may benefit from this collection, but I was slightly sickened by the thought that they would need to.

Once the collection was complete, the catheter was removed. To my surprise, this was done bedside by the nurse simply clipping the stitches that were holding it in place and then quickly pulling it out. Due to the size of the hole left by the catheter, pressure needed to be applied directly to the area for several minutes, and then a large bandage was placed over the top of it. We left the hospital later that afternoon and were extremely excited of the promise of staying home together for about five days before coming back in for round three.

Chapter Ten

After Patiently Enduring, We Obtain the Promise

(Hebrews 6:15)

*O*ur time together passed far too quickly, as seemed to be the case those days, and we were due back at the hospital before we knew it. While no chemo is easy or fun, we were informed that these next four rounds of chemo held more intense side effects and would overall be more difficult for Lexi's body to handle. In each round, Lexi was given two types of chemo, with each chemo holding its own horrors. This round, Lexi would be getting cisplatin—commonly recognized as the most nauseating chemo used—and etoposide—a chemo known to actually cause cancer later in life. Trust me, the irony that they use a medication to cure cancer that can actually end up causing cancer was not lost on me.

When your child's life is threatened, you find yourself in a difficult position. In any other situation, you would avoid these medications at all costs, but instead we found ourselves signing consent forms. Lexi needed this medication to get her through this battle, even if it meant she might face another one down the road. Many well-meaning people told us of multiple holistic methods that would be far less damaging. In some cases, they even knew of someone who had been personally healed by the method.

I lean on holistic medication for coughs, foot powder, and even headaches, but when it came to the knowledge that our daughter's life was in jeopardy, we wanted the most guaranteed treatment plan we could find. We wanted medication that had been tested and proven by thousands of people for decades. This meant that the side effects came with it. Every person who is battling cancer needs to find their own approach to dealing with this monster, but as we prayed, we knew the path we needed to take, even if that path was laced with mines.

The side effects had been discussed, papers handed to me, and the nurse walked in cloaked in the chemo protection garb. She hung the medications on the IV pole that Lexi would be chained to for the next week and checked her vitals. Not thirty minutes after the toxin started flowing into her veins did we discover that cisplatin had gained its reputation for a reason. Lexi's body began retching uncontrollably. It was apparent that this week would be far more difficult than we had prepared for. The hours crept by, and Lexi's body continued to try to expel the poison that was being pumped into it.

Lexi was already getting the four standard anti-nausea medications that she had been getting with the previous rounds. However, it was clearly not enough. Doctors came in and added Dexamethasone, Olanzapine, and a Scopolamine patch to the regimen of Zofran, Benadryl, Phenergan, and Ativan. A small bottle containing two cotton balls was brought in as well. Peppermint oil is known to have natural anti-nausea properties, so oil had been dripped on each cotton ball. With these added measures, Lexi was able to go as much as fifteen minutes in between vomiting. Occasionally she would be able to fall into a restless sleep in my arms with the aid of all of the medications. We were grateful for these short periods of rest that allowed her body to sometimes go as long as thirty minutes without vomiting.

The days turned into nights and back into days without us knowing. Each day bore the same exhaustion as the one before as I lay next to my daughter, praying for some relief. In just three days' time, she had lost five more pounds, bringing her five-foot, seven-inch frame down to only 105 pounds. I held her and watched the life-saving poison being pumped into her weak body as the hours passed. She awoke once and feebly said, "Mom, is it Tuesday morning already?"

"No, honey, it is Thursday night." Cancer was quite literally stealing days from her that she wouldn't get back.

"How can I help you, honey? What can I do?" I knew I was grasping at straws, but I wanted nothing more than to take this from her.

"Just hold me, Mama," she softly responded. "It helps when I'm in your arms." So together we sat on the small couch that doubled as my makeshift bed, and I cradled my fifteen-year-old daughter as we both silently prayed for this trial to pass.

Lexi's days were spent in a dim room, wishing the time would pass quicker. She woke for a few moments at a time, only to try to fall asleep again. Messages were sent from family and friends to offer support and encouragement, and I would read them to her as she drifted in and out of consciousness. Previous rounds paled in comparison to what this week had done to her.

I was struggling to process how hard Lexi had been hit. This was only the end of round three. We were only halfway through our first step of treatment, and her body had already taken such a beating. The thought of how much more she would have to endure made me physically ill. I recited my concerns to Kris, and he brought a new perspective to my mind. He said that cancer is like a really good boxing match.

Each round, the challenger gets knocked down, just to get up again. Each round, the body becomes weaker and sustains more damage, but the mental resolve to win grows. For while the physical strength of the challenger seems to be dwindling, her mental reserve is building.

The challenger barely has time to stand, showing that she is competent to continue with the fight before getting hit again, knocking her already-damaged body lower than it was before. She commands herself to stand again, and the fight continues.

Finally, the match ends, and the challenger, barely able to stand, lifts her head in triumph. The marks of the battle will be carried throughout her life as a physical reminder of the anguish she endured. She will look to those scars—both seen and unseen—as reminders that when she could have stayed down, she chose to stand and fight.

Throughout my life, when I had been faced with difficult trials, I would often pray for the strength I needed to get through the trial. However, there are things we will have to endure in this life that no amount of mortal strength will ever be enough to get us through. I knew I would never be strong enough to watch my child suffer through what she would have to in order to be whole again.

Instead, I prayed for endurance. I prayed that we would be able to endure this trial with faith and grace. I prayed that we would have the endurance to remain true to who we were and who we were striving to be. I prayed that we would be able to endure with humility and gratitude whatever trials would come our way, and even continue to look for the goodness in the world around us. I prayed that no matter how long it took, we would have the endurance to never give up—ever. I prayed that long after my physical and emotional strength had been depleted, I would have the endurance to carry on. Once again I felt strength beyond my own buoy me up, and I took comfort in knowing that I was not alone in praying for our little family.

The week had finally come to an end, and we were able to once again be reunited with Kris, Cam, Liv, and Aleah. The strength we found in one another rejuvenated our spirits and filled our souls. As we drove home, we felt grateful to be done with yet another round of chemo, and we were looking forward to putting this draining week behind us. We pulled into our driveway and honked the horn. All of the kids came running out. This had become a tradition over the past few months. My heart always swelled at seeing how much joy my children found in being together. It was an opportunity that they no longer took for granted. I took a deep breath and realized that we had done it. We had made it through a week that was unlike anything I could imagine—a week that would always be considered one of our most difficult. However, while we were at a low point, there were others planning a way to lift our spirits back to the top.

Lexi's drill team, their parents and families, her coaches, and the members of our community had worked tirelessly to plan a dance concert on behalf of our family. It would take place the day after we got home from the hospital. We loaded up the car with the kids and all of the necessary supplies for a night out on the town and headed over to the school. The concert was titled "Tonight We Dance Alexis Strong," and it featured drill teams and dance teams from all over the state. We had heard that this concert was being organized, but we were in complete awe at the turnout it had produced.

Just before the concert began, Lexi's coaches greeted me with a warm hug and said, "Em, we want you guys to walk down Blood Alley to start the concert."

Holding each of their hands I looked at them. "It has to be all of us," I said. "It needs to be all of my kids."

"Of course," Natalie responded.

"We were planning on it," Sara chimed in.

The time approached, and the gym doors opened. I saw Lexi's drill team lined up in two parallel lines, just like they had been on the sides of my cracked driveway. The MC for the night began reading the story of Alexis, her journey thus far, and what else she would need to endure. I grabbed Liv's hand in one of mine and Cam's in the other. It was as much for me as it was for them. We needed each other. If we had any chance of getting through this, it would be together. Cam grabbed Lexi's hand as she took Kris's. Kris held to Aleah's hand, and we stood as we listened to what our family had gone through and what we would need to go through in order to survive. At the conclusion of Lexi's bio, we began walking hand in hand through Blood Alley. Every person in attendance stood to show their love and support for our family.

Once again, my tears spilled over, but this time Livi reached her hand up and wiped them away lovingly. Her green eyes sparkled, and she smiled brightly at me. I ventured a glance at Aleah. She loved the attention and that people were applauding for her family. She smiled and waved while holding her daddy's hand. I looked to Kris, whose gaze was on Lexi, making sure she was okay. She was wearing a radiant smile and carrying herself with grace beyond her years. My eyes fell to Cam, and then my heart fell as well. There was no excitement in his eyes or broad smile on his face. He knew why they were standing and understood better than most what we were facing. He walked solemnly, prepared to fight this battle by his sister's side.

It was a night that shone brightly after such a dark week; a night that illuminated our heavy spirits and filled our souls with much-needed light. We had told our children that we were not alone in this battle. As we walked hand in hand across a crowded gymnasium in our hometown, they saw visual evidence that we truly had an army behind us. It was a night that our spirits needed and our hearts would never forget.

Chapter Eleven

I'm Filled with Charity, Which Is Everlasting Love

(Moroni 8:17)

*B*efore we knew it, we found ourselves at the hospital, ready to conquer round four of chemo. Hospitals are notorious for not having any cell service. Add this to the fact that there are always medical professionals coming in and out of your room with new information, and when they are telling you what they are injecting into the tube that leads to your daughter's heart and the effects it will have, you tend to give the doctors and nurses your undivided attention. So, rather than try to carry on a conversation where only every other word gets through, I generally opted to text while we were inpatient. We had gotten settled into our surroundings, and the premedication had begun for round four. The nurse had just left the room when my phone rang in my hand. I didn't recognize the number, but something told me that this was one call I needed to take, so I answered it.

The woman on the line said that her name was Teresa Whitehead and that she was the CEO of City Wide Mortgage. I greeted her, not fully understanding why the CEO of a major corporation would be calling my cell phone. She went on to say that our family had been nominated several times to receive a home makeover. I asked her if she was sure that she had the right number. "Is this Emily Gould—Alexis Gould's mother?" My heart stopped, and I slowly confirmed her question. She again stated that we had been nominated for a home makeover. My mind reeled as she spoke. We had already received an outpouring of love and support from our family, friends, and community. Surely this was too much. I was speechless, and I could do nothing more than listen.

Teresa told me that in lieu of a Christmas party, their company had decided to begin a tradition the year before known as "Makeovers from the Heart," in which they remodeled a room or two for a few houses of people who were going through difficult times. "Is there a time I can meet with you and Kris at your home for a walkthrough?" she asked. I told her that Lexi and I were in the hospital but gave her Kris's information to set up a meeting. Immediately after hanging up with Teresa, I called Kris. He was stunned. Neither of us could understand how in the midst of their busy schedules so many people would take time from their lives to try to lighten our loads in this manner. We were in awe.

We lived in an older home in an older community. It was nothing spectacular, but it was ours, and we were content. We updated and did repairs as they came and as time and money allowed, but they often took a back seat to more pressing matters. With our lives taking the turn they had, we were in no position financially or any other way to focus on our home at that time. Others had looked for a way to help, to fill a need we hadn't even recognized in order to show love and support to our family. Our hearts were again humbled to feel the genuine love and generosity of those around us.

Teresa arranged a time, and she and a few of her associates met with Kris at our home. She did a walkthrough and told Kris that they would need to discuss some things but were hoping to be able to redo our bathroom. This was our next big project, one that we knew couldn't be put off much longer, and my heart swelled knowing that this would take something so major off of our plate.

A few days passed, and Kris called me at the hospital. "Are you sitting down?" he asked. A sense of disbelief seemed to travel from his voice through the phone line. "I just got off the phone with Teresa."

"Okay . . ." I said, waiting for him to continue.

There was a long pause, followed by, "They want to remodel our entire house—everything."

"Are you sure?" I said with incredulity. "Are you sure that's what they said? Everything?"

"Everything," he confirmed. "She said that there was an outpouring from friends and members of the community who are willing to be a part of the project, many of them donating their labor for free. They want us to pack our entire house up. They will get us storage units and a place to stay for about three weeks while they completely remodel our entire house."

I could tell from his voice that he was having the same thoughts I was. "It's too much," I said. "It's just too much."

You would think that upon hearing the news that someone is going to give you a brand-new home, a person would shed tears of joy. However, happiness was not the source of my leaky tear ducts. Guilt, sadness, and sorrow accompanied this beautiful gift. The guilt came in knowing that there were other children, other families, out there suffering and fighting this battle just as we were. Were they not just as deserving, if not more so, than our family? Had they not had to endure the same angst, sadness, and sorrow? Had they not suffered heartache and desperation? Why us and not them?

The sadness and sorrow stemmed from knowing why our family was nominated. It wasn't because we won a contest or an award. We were nominated because our daughter had cancer. We were nominated because people knew that this experience would bring with it more than we could comprehend, more than our hearts could bear, and they were looking to ease our pain in any way possible.

I spoke with a dear friend about the inner turmoil I was facing. He offered a wise perspective. "Em, there are many people, not just you and Kris, who would gladly take this pain from Lexi, from your family, but we can't. This is something that we can do. We can't save your family from what you'll go through, but we will do whatever we can to make the pain more bearable." I listened and tried to humble my heavy heart. He continued, "Lexi being diagnosed and the way people are reaching out to help is bigger than just your family. Emily, people are realizing that there are still good people in the world that want to help others out. Don't hide that. Let them help."

It was humbling to recognize that while you have nothing to give in return, there are still those who would do all they could to carry your load. Kris and I talked about it, and when we got home from the hospital, we talked together as a family. The choice was reached and plans were made. It was decided that we would move out of our home the weekend after Thanksgiving and hopefully move back just in time for Christmas.

The following weeks brought a sense of excitement that filled our lives. I had been thankful for the temporal blessing of having our home repaired, but had vastly underestimated the emotional and psychological healing it would offer. We found ourselves with a new project that was not centered around cancer at all. We took to packing up our house and keeping ourselves busy with anything that was not medically based. Of course, cancer did not take a back seat entirely. There were still clinic appointments to be kept, home health-care visits to have, medications, and so on. However, cancer was not center stage right now. Our kids had something else to focus on, something exciting happening in their life to counteract the negative. They were told that they could visit Pinterest and choose some ideas of color schemes for their rooms. For the first time since diagnosis, someone was doing something equally for each of them, and my heart could not have been more grateful.

Slowly, all of our belongings were moved into the provided storage containers. Everything we would no longer need was donated to those in our neighborhood who could use it. The day before demolition was scheduled, Cam asked if he could punch a hole in his wall. Of course, my first mom thought was, *No! Are you crazy? We don't punch holes in the walls!* Luckily, I caught myself and realized that we had a once-in-a-lifetime opportunity here. "Sure!" I said. "Just let me come and watch!" I went down to his room and made sure he was lined up so as not to hit a stud. He expelled some built up rage by punching through the wall. I don't think he realized it would be a little more difficult than in the movies.

"Mom, do you think you can do it?" he said.

"Of course I can!" I replied with a false confidence that he luckily didn't pick up on. I balled my fist and slammed it through the wall. The wall broke beneath the pressure, and I pulled my hand out of the sheetrock. I looked at him and shrugged like it was no big deal and then went upstairs to simultaneously laugh and cry at my stupidity. There was no question about it. It definitely hurt more than they let on in the movies.

The day of demolition arrived, and we were invited to our house to see it take place. To our astonishment, far more than just a few people showed up to help. Teresa was there, along with the owner of City Wide Mortgage and many of their employees. Lexi's drill team and their families had also shown up, along with a few young men from the high school football team. The plan was now in full motion. We spent Thanksgiving together and then moved into our temporary home—an extended-stay hotel just a few minutes from our house—just in time for Lexi to begin her next round of chemo the following Monday.

As we were unpacking our week's worth of luggage, we were surprised to learn that this round of chemo would require her to only stay inpatient for four days. This would be our shortest hospital stay yet! The following days were no walk in the park, but compared to what she had endured, we found ourselves grateful for no major setbacks. Exhausted yet appreciative that this round was not as damaging as the last, we brought Lexi home to the hotel to recover and wait for the next round.

The newness of the hotel had not yet worn off, and the kids were excited to tell us all about the swimming pool every night and the hot chocolate every morning. Kris had already gotten them into a routine, and they were thoroughly enjoying their new surroundings. We had been given two large rooms that were next to each other. It was decided that Cam, Liv, and Leah would share one room—Cam having his own bed and the girls bunking together. Kris and I were in the other room, and Lexi would sleep on the pull-out sofa in our room in case she needed something in the middle of the night. We spent the night decorating a Christmas tree that some dear friends had brought to us and just enjoying the thought of spending the holiday season in our home away from home for the next few weeks.

After showing me at least five times where each of their beds were located, Cam and the girls finally fell asleep. Lexi was having some discomfort, so we gave her some medication in addition to her nightly pharmacy and kissed her good night as well. I climbed into bed and contentedly fell asleep, knowing everything was as it should be. Morning came, and Kris and I helped the kids get ready for school. To my surprise, Lexi was already awake, and pain was evident in her eyes.

"I've been up all night, but I didn't want to wake you guys, because I knew how tired you must be."

"Sis, we've talked about this. I'm not going to be able to sleep at all if I don't think you'll wake me up when you need me. Please wake me up if you're not able to sleep so we can take care of whatever you need."

She agreed and then continued explaining what was wrong. "It's just hard for me to breathe, and I'm having a really sharp pain on the right side of my chest." She tried to walk herself to the bathroom, just ten feet away from her makeshift bed, but she was too weak. Something was horribly wrong. My stomach dropped.

We asked a few more questions about the intensity of her pain and considered that what she was describing was possibly some type of reaction to the chemo she had just finished. I wasn't even sure if that was a possibility, but I'd recently learned that many things existed that I would never have dreamt possible. Kris and I decided that it would be best if he dropped the kids off at school and I drove Lexi back to the clinic immediately. We said our good-byes. I kissed Kris and my kids and told them that we would be home from clinic by the time they made it back from school.

We had been home only eighteen short hours, and the last thing I wanted to do was stay at the hospital any longer than we needed to. I assumed that we would stay in clinic long enough for them to give her something to help with the reaction and we would be on our way. I should've known that nothing was that simple with cancer.

We drove to the hospital and went straight to the clinic. Lexi was checked in, and I helped her to a room. She was becoming noticeably weaker than she was just a few hours ago, and I was doing my best to control the flashbacks that were flooding my mind of the night we came to the ER. The doctors came to our room and examined Lexi. The pain she described, coupled with her behavior, was enough for them to order an x-ray. It revealed nothing, so an ultrasound was done. Again, nothing. There were no other indications of what was going on, but after consulting with one another, they reached the conclusion that given the aggressiveness of Lexi's cancer and her history with pneumonia, they weren't willing to take any risks. "We want to admit Lexi just overnight for monitoring," the doctor said. We agreed, not out of compliance, but understanding that it was what was best for Lexi.

Lexi's wheelchair was gingerly pushed from the clinic to the ICS double doors and through them to our room. The pain was getting worse, but Lex just wanted to go home. "Mom, let me just tell them that it's not that bad. I just want to go home. I miss our family. Maybe it will just go away on its own." My heart hurt. I knew she didn't want to stay, but I knew she wasn't healthy enough to go home. I stopped walking.

I looked into her eyes and said, "If you can walk out of here unassisted, we will leave right now." Tears filled her eyes and mine, because we both knew she wasn't well enough to do that. I called Kris and told him the news—he was a single dad again, at least for the night.

The next day brought more pain and more tests. They decided to do another x-ray to see if perhaps something had been missed the previous day. More labs were drawn and tests were run in hopes of finding any indication as to what may be causing her pain. We had just returned to her room from more imaging. As I was helping her into her bed, her forehead brushed my cheek. My mom-dar (that's a mom radar—a completely real thing) went off, telling me that she had a fever. Upon my request, the nurse took her temperature and found that she was running a fever of 102.7 degrees Fahrenheit. She called the team and brought in some Tylenol. Not an hour later, the team came in. The results from the day's imaging had come back.

Once again, Lexi had pneumonia, but in addition to that, she was fighting off pleural effusion, and her labs returned, showing that she had contracted multiple viruses. The pain was being caused by the fluid and infection in the lining of her lungs. It had been hidden in previous imaging by her tumor but was very visible on the images taken that day. Her counts had already dropped to 0.0, meaning that she had absolutely nothing to fight off any illness or infection. She was being attacked and had no way to defend herself. The doctors explained that because her immune system was currently compromised, she would not only need to stay in the hospital, but she would also be confined to her room.

This sentence was to be carried out until her counts came up, her fevers broke, her pneumonia and pleural effusion were gone, and her body had conquered the viruses and infections. A procedure would also need to be done to drain the fluid in her lungs. There was no time frame given. We were at the mercy of her damaged body and how fast it could fight to recover.

When we came to the hospital the day before, I was expecting a short visit with the possibility of some tests and imaging to ease the mind of an overprotective mother. I had helped my kids get ready and kissed them good-bye with the intention of eating dinner together that night. Now I didn't know the next time I would have that opportunity. Even more heart wrenching was the knowledge that it was flu season. That may not hold much weight in a healthy world, but because of the risks that the flu poses to people with no immune system, there were seasonal restrictions enforced for visitors at the hospital during that time. Those restrictions extended to anyone who was sick and anyone under the age of twelve. This meant that for an indefinite period of time, my family would not be able to sit in the same room together. Lexi was not the only one feeling a pain in her chest that night.

The procedure was done the following day, but the other infections and viruses had stepped up their game, making Lexi feel worse than before. In addition to this, the "normal" side effects of chemo were beginning to manifest. Cancer cells are fast growing—like hair and skin cells. Chemo cannot distinguish between the good cells and the bad cells, so it works by attacking all fast-growing cells. This is why patients going through chemo lose their hair.

Losing your hair is not a physically painful process, but losing the lining of the skin in your mouth is. Mucusitis—more commonly known as mouth sores—is perhaps one of the most painful temporary side effects of chemo, and Lexi was beginning to experience them worse than ever. The pain was so intense that Lexi wasn't able to eat or even speak for days on end. While having a teenager that can't talk may sound ideal, it is not quite all it's cracked up to be. Communication is important, so Lex and I got extremely good at charades.

Seeing the impact that these common viruses were having on Lexi's weakened body reminded me of the wonderment of the human body. When functioning properly, our bodies have the ability to fight off disease and heal with little to no effort. The infections and illnesses that were keeping Lexi hostage in a sterile room would have been nothing more than an inconvenience or a few sick days to anyone else. On a daily basis, we are protected from dangers we don't even know exist. It is only when our bodies are compromised, when we are in a weakened state, that we understand how truly vulnerable we are. We are quick to complain about feeling under the weather, but do we truly appreciate the fact that our bodies, in most cases, can fully rejuvenate and renew themselves when functioning properly? We are literal miracles.

Chapter Twelve

Men Are That They Might Have Joy
(2 Nephi 2:25)

*T*he days passed slowly and uneventfully. In order to help her defenseless body heal, Lexi was started on a regimen that consisted of multiple anti-viral, anti-fungal antibiotics and anti-nausea medication. And, of course, pain medication to try to ease the suffering brought on by the mouth sores. Each of these medications had to be delivered intravenously, because the mouth sores had extended down her throat and taken away her ability to swallow. TPN was started to try to avoid further weight loss. Sleep was induced by the medication and encouraged by the doctors as a way to let her body rest and apply all energy to the purpose of healing.

The brief moments that she was awake were filled doing things that would pass the time. Most of the games, activities, and crafts at the hospital are geared to children of a much younger age, so Lexi and I had to learn to create our own fun. Being confined to a small room drastically limits what a person can do for excitement, and being indescribably sick limits them further. So I had to get creative. I had ventured out to the cafeteria one afternoon and looked out the window to realize that it was snowing. It wasn't just an ordinary storm either. It was a beautiful snow—the kind that consists of big flakes that even grown men try to catch on their tongue. I watched it fall and yearned for a day filled with laughter and sledding with my family.

I continued on to the cafeteria thinking about the snow and how different our reality was now. Lexi was in a hospital room. Even if she wanted to, she would not be able to go play in the snow. Cam would likely still take the opportunity to build a hill in the backyard for Liv and Leah to slide down, but I wouldn't be there to watch them do it, to see their red noses as they came in, to make them hot chocolate and listen to how much fun they had. That was not our life right now. Sadness is a tricky emotion. It is one that needs to be felt and expressed, but if not contained, it has the ability to quickly taint any situation.

We were in a difficult circumstance. That was easy to recognize. I had taken the time to feel sad, and now it was time to look for opportunities that wouldn't be available in other situations. I quickly got my lunch and grabbed two extra food containers. I was grinning like a toddler who had just found an unsupervised bag of goldfish crackers. I passed a door that was unlocked and headed outside in my T-shirt and leggings. I walked only a few feet from the door, bent down, and collected snow in each of the containers. I hurried back to our room as quickly as I could.

I often ate in our room so that I was there in case Lexi needed something. So, seeing me walk in with food containers was not a surprise to her. The goofy grin on my face is what caught her attention. "I have something for you," I said.

She still wasn't able to speak. Instead she just quizzically raised her non-existent eyebrows.

"Guess what it is!" I said enthusiastically. She attempted a smile through swollen cheeks and shrugged her shoulders. I then opened the first container and said, "Today we are going to build a snowman!" She made a noise that was the closest thing I had heard to a laugh in a week, and my heart leapt.

Maybe we didn't have the opportunity to do all of the things we had always done, but we could take the opportunity to do things we had never done before. I grabbed a pair of rubber gloves from the box on the wall and handed them to Lex, hoping to keep her hands from getting too cold. She put them on excitedly. The next twenty minutes was spent building and accessorizing our small snowman. He was then placed in the food container on the small table in our room. Lexi gestured to him when the nurses came in and had me recount the story of how he got there. Throughout the day, we watched as little by little he turned into a puddle of water.

It quickly became my mission to do something each day to bring joy into our hospital room in some new and unexpected way. The feeling became contagious, and soon we found new things to laugh about every day. On one particular morning, we heard a knock at our door. A young man entered and asked Lexi if she would like to play bingo with the other patients. Lexi was still unable to leave her room, let alone have any contact with other patients. So, instead of gathering in a room to play bingo, everyone wishing to play simply tuned in to the same TV station at a particular time. The young man explained the concept, handed her a paper, and told her that she could win a prize for playing. Lexi had been given the opportunity to play many times before but had not felt up to it. Today wasn't much different.

We thanked him and took the paper, and he left. A few minutes later, I left for the cafeteria for my mandated outing. When I came back, I found Lexi resting and some hair clips sitting on the sink next to the door in her room. Aware of the fact that I was the only person in the room with hair and they were not my clips, I found myself a little confused.

When Lexi awoke, I motioned to the hair clips. "Where did these come from?" I asked. What tried to be a large smile crossed Lexi's face, and her shoulders slightly shook as a snicker softly escaped her torn-up mouth.

Through gritted teeth she responded, "Those are my bingo prize!"

I stifled a laugh. "They brought you, a patient on the cancer floor, hair clips?" Her grin widened slightly as she nodded her head. "Were you just sleeping when they got here? Were you just cuddled under the blankets? Did they not see you?" I asked, assuming that there was no way that someone would knowingly bring hair clips to a bald teenage girl. Despite the pain, her smile broadened and she spoke through gritted teeth.

"He came in and talked to me. He said he had my prize for winning bingo—even though I didn't play—and asked where I wanted them set. I pointed to the sink, and he put them down and left."

I couldn't contain my laughter anymore. "So you are saying that a young man came in, looked at you, talked to you, and then left hair clips for you?" Her shoulders shook with laughter as she held her cheeks in pain. I joined in the laughter, and as our nurse entered the room, Lexi motioned for me to reiterate the story for the nurse's enjoyment. The nurse asked all of the same questions I did, and Lex just sat on the bed doing her best to contain her smile and minimize the pain from the mouth sores.

Later that afternoon, we were heading to the tub room. Each patient room has a shower, but if a patient wants to take a bath, they have to schedule the tub room. Lexi preferred baths to showers, because they helped ease muscle cramps and pain, so our nurse made sure that the tub room had been cleaned specifically for her. By this time, word of her bingo prize had spread around the floor. So, as we walked down the hall, IV pole in tow, many comments and laughs were had between Lex and the nurses on exactly how she would use her newly claimed prize. Clip-on earrings and brooches were among the top suggestions, both of which were modeled with the utmost exaggeration.

We entered the tub room, and the familiar scent of bleach filled my nose. We hadn't taken but a few steps when Lexi stopped dead in her tracks. A large smile played on her lips and again her swollen face showed the threat of laughter. I followed her gaze and found that there, on top of her freshly folded towels, was a brush, a bottle of hair detangler, and a few small bottles of shampoo and conditioner. I laughed right out loud. I poked my head out to see several nurses at the charge desk laughing hysterically.

"You have no idea how hard we had to look to find that stuff up here!" One nurse said.

"We had everyone searching for it!" Another piped up.

"We just really wanted to add to her hair care accessories!" A third nurse chimed in. It felt good to genuinely laugh at such an ironic situation.

However, Lexi is not one to be outdone when it comes to jokes. After her bath she took a towel, wrapped it around her bald head as if she had hair, and paraded down the halls of the cancer unit amidst the laughter of nurses. She did her best with her aching mouth to thank them for the hair care products and told them that her hair felt better than it had in months. The loss of hair is a traumatic experience for many cancer patients and can be a very sensitive subject. Lexi loved her hair and missed it terribly, but she believed that you could either laugh or cry at the situation, and she really loved to laugh.

The fact that our family could not spend time together in the ways we always had, meant that we had to work harder to make sure that our relationships were stronger than ever. Kris would bring the kids up to visit as often as possible. He would sit with Lex while she rested, or visit with her if she was up for it. Meanwhile, Liv and Leah would go with me to the cafeteria to play games. Cam rotated his time between visiting with me and spending time with Lex. Visiting time always started by walking to the University of Utah hospital and riding the escalator up to the second floor just to ride it back down again. This activity was generally followed by dinner or treats in the cafeteria, card games, and, from time to time, a trip to the gift shop to look around.

During these special times, I reveled in their storytelling as my kids caught me up on everything that was happening at school and at home. They would then ask about Lexi, and I would give my most honest, age-appropriate answer. Although the topics varied, one question was asked every time.

"Mom, when can you and Lexi come home?" The hardest questions are always the ones you can't answer.

I couldn't give them a false hope, so rather than a date, I gave them the parameters that needed to be met. We then could track our progress, and they could focus on the goal rather than the date.

On one particular visit, Cam opted to stay with Kris and Lexi. The girls and I had just finished up in the cafeteria, so hand in hand, we walked into the gift shop and began looking around. They loved to see the encouraging words on the plaques, the stuffed animals, and the uplifting cards. One card in particular caught Livi's eye. It had a picture on the front of the card of three girls with their arms around each other's backs.

"Mom, look!" Liv said. "This looks like me, Lexi, and Leah! Can we get this and write Lexi a note for you to take up to her?" I smiled and nodded. We bought the card and headed to a table in the cafeteria. I gave Livi a pen, and she proceeded to draw a boy stick figure with his arm around his sisters. She held it up to show me her masterpiece. "This is Cam. Now we can all be together." My heart swelled as I realized that even when my children were not able to physically be in the same room, they would always be in each other's hearts.

Yes, it was hard not being together. But how many times do we share the same space with someone, yet our thoughts and feelings are miles away? Closeness in relationships is not based on physical proximity. It is much deeper than that, and to my great relief, our children understood this concept. Tears filled my eyes and spilled onto my cheeks. Aleah lovingly smiled and wiped them with her small hand. They didn't ask why I cried anymore. They just comforted me when the tears could not be contained.

Our visit came to an end, and it was time to head back to the crying couches to meet Kris and Cam so they could all get to bed and wake up in time for school the next morning. The closer we got to the rendezvous point, the tighter our hands grasped one another's, as if somehow this desperate attempt at holding on would be enough to not have to let go. The whimsical chatter slowly quieted, and we fell into silence, knowing that our time was coming to an end. Kris and Cam were waiting for the girls, and I looked to see the familiar tears once again on my children's faces. I strived to wipe them away without shedding too many of my own. We talked about how hard this was and what needed to happen before we could come home. It was the same parting scene every time. Cry, talk, loves, extra loves for Lexi, repeat. It was a heart-wrenching déjà vu that would replay in my mind during the sleepless nights.

The hours turned into days, and days into weeks. Lexi's mouth sores were still painful but began to slowly heal. Her cough lessened, and her fevers stopped. Now came the waiting game. Her ANC would have to recover before we could leave. Each night we would pray that tomorrow would be the day that her labs showed improvement, and each morning we were told, "No change yet, but we should see something any day now." We would anxiously await the dawning of a new day to hear the morning report that accompanied it only to learn that there was yet to be an end in sight. Christmas was creeping closer and closer, but my heart was heavier than ever.

I have always enjoyed learning, and I like to think that there is something to learn in every situation. I don't believe that we are left to suffer or experience heartache for no apparent reason. I believe with my whole heart that we are given experiences for the purpose of growing. However, I found myself struggling with what I could learn from the scenario we currently found ourselves in. My heart was in a constant state of prayer and pleading. What was to be learned from this? What lesson came in children's heartache? What was to be learned from keeping my family apart?

I thought back over the previous weeks. My mind recalled the many times I had really felt that we would be heading home the next day, only to be disappointed in learning that no change had been made. We were stuck—indefinitely.

I figured that the lesson I was to learn was patience; however, I wasn't really sure that patience was actually the lesson. Patience is the scapegoat lesson I tend to fall on when my prayers have not been answered in the manner or timing that I think is best. In this particular case, it sounded pretty accurate, so I stuck with it. Patience—that was my lesson. I was to learn patience, and I really prayed that I could learn it quickly so we could go home. I tried to alter my prayers and accept that things happened in the Lord's time. I tried to focus not on the days spent apart but the time we got together and how very precious it was. I did my best to exhibit every bit of patience my exhausted heart could muster. I was so focused on quickly learning patience that I almost missed the real lesson that was before me.

Lexi's counts (meaning her white blood cells and absolute neutrophil count in this instance) had been at 0.0 for the past couple of weeks. A healthy body generally registers anywhere in the 4.3 to 10.8 range for WBC and 1.5 to 8.0 for ANC. For the past week, her labs were indicating that at any day we would see a change indicating that her immune system was beginning to make a comeback. The general pattern is that the WBC count will come up first, followed by the ANC. But her WBC did not seem to be in any hurry to regenerate. Day after day we waited with no change—then one morning it happened. Lexi's WBC went to 0.1. We were elated at that small victory but were reminded to not be discouraged if the labs the following day showed that her counts had fallen again, since this was a common occurrence with count recovery. Either way, we were just grateful for the change in counts and the promise it held that we were heading in the right direction.

For the next three days, her WBC stayed at 0.1, and I found myself overjoyed that it didn't falter. Her body wasn't strong enough to progress much further yet, but it wasn't willing to back down. On the fourth day, her WBC raised to 0.2. By our reaction, you would've thought that she had just won the Olympic Gold medal in count recovery. Her body fought so hard, not only to maintain the 0.1 count, but to also find the strength to push itself just that little bit more. It was then that I understood that patience was not the sole lesson I needed to be taught. Rather, I needed to be reminded the importance of not overlooking the small victories in life.

It was now December 22. Lexi's medication was switched from IV to oral in hopes that we would be able to make it home for Christmas just the day before. "You know Lex," the nurse said, "even if you do have to stay, Christmas in the hospital is not too bad. They feel really bad for kids that have to stay here, so you'll get spoiled. They bring kids so many presents and really try to make it so fun. There are definitely worse places you could be for Christmas."

Lex smiled. "The only thing I want for Christmas is to be home with my family. I want to be with my brother and sisters and my dad and mom, all of us together. I haven't hugged my sisters in almost a month, and I want to be with them." The nurse smiled and promised that they would do their best to get her home.

The next day, the doctors came in. "Lexi, do you want to go home today?!" I think they were as excited to deliver the Christmas news as Lexi was to hear it.

"Really?!"

"It will be later today, but we will start the process, and you can sleep in your own bed tonight."

"This is the best Christmas present ever!!" Lexi said.

"What are you hoping to get for Christmas?" The doctors asked, clearly in a more talkative mood because of the season.

"I don't need anything. I just want to be home with my family. Nothing else matters." My heart was bursting. Our prayers had been heard and answered. We would be together again soon, all of us. I looked at Lex, and she grinned mischievously. "Mom, can you find me a box?"

Chapter Thirteen

There Was Peace and Exceedingly Great Joy

(Helaman 3:32)

*L*exi quickly told me her plan and was so excited about it that she could barely contain herself. In the midst of paperwork and packing up a month's worth of living space and decorations, we found a large box. I called Kris and told him that we had officially been discharged and that we were heading back to the hotel. He was in on Lexi's plan and had all of the kids go into the adjoining room that they had been staying in to watch TV. Over the previous few days, we had updated Cam, Liv, and Leah on Lexi's progress but did not have the heart to assure them that we would be home by Christmas.

We made it back to the hotel, where Kris met us at the elevators and helped us to the room. We were too excited to unpack right then, so we carried only the box with us to the room. Kris then stood guard while Lexi climbed into the box and I wrapped it with shiny paper. I knew that my presence would spoil any surprise, so I asked Kris to record them opening the present, and I hid behind the door leading into the bedroom.

Kris got the kids from the adjoining room, and once they saw the gift, the three of them attacked the box, eager to see its contents. Excitement and joy lit their faces as the box opened to reveal their sister inside. "LEXI!" they simultaneously shouted, and then they tried—not to help her out of the box (that would take too much pre-cious time)—to climb into the box to hug her.

"Was that a good surprise?" I asked as I came out from behind the door.

"Mom!" They jumped out of the box and wrapped their arms around me. All of the sleepless nights, the worrying, wondering, and heartache-induced pain disappeared in that moment. We were together, and nothing else mattered.

While Lexi had been working hard to make it home, many nights, weekends, and long hours were sacrificed by Teresa from City Wide Mortgage, her team, and our friends in hopes of getting us back into our home in time for Christmas. The walk through of our house had originally been scheduled for December 20 but had been postponed a few days in hopes that we would all be able to see our new house together for the first time. We were together at the hotel for only an hour before we got the call that we could go see our new home.

We drove to the same address we had for the past thirteen years, but things looked so different. A small group of people had gathered for the unveiling, and I hugged Teresa, now a dear friend, as we walked to the front door. We went room by room, and the transformation was breathtaking. Each of my kids took time to discover their new living space that had been personally created for them. My kitchen was beautiful, and we now had two bathrooms instead of one. Framed snapshots of our family were found scat-tered throughout the house, making it feel more like our space. It was more beautiful than I had imagined, but the biggest blessing was yet to come.

I walked downstairs to mine and Kris's room. I turned to look at my dresser, and my breath caught. I slowly reached my hand out, and a tear rolled down my cheek. There on my new dresser were displayed some of my most precious possessions. It was not jewelry or expensive décor. It was the flowers that my kids had made for me every year for Mother's day or my birthday, the ones made from their hands. My fingers touched the flower-shaped cardboard that Lexi had spent hours coloring. I smiled as I touched the flowers made out of the shape of Cam's hands when they were still smaller than mine. My smile continued to grow as my eyes fell to the flowers made from pipe cleaner from Olivia, and the ones made out of scrapbook paper that fit Aleah's personality. There are some memories that cancer doesn't get to touch.

We officially moved back into our home, all of us together as a family, on Christmas Eve. That night, despite each of my babies having their own brand new rooms to sleep in, all of them slept together in the same room, just like they had every year. On Christmas Day, Cam and Lex woke up and made the rest of us breakfast in bed, just like they had every year for the past five-plus years. While they were making breakfast, Cam looked at Lex and smiled. Later that day, Lex told me of their tender conversation.

"You know what, Flex?"

"What?" she said, smiling at the nickname he had adopted for her.

"I'm really glad you are home. I really missed you," he said.

"Me too," Lexi replied.

"You know, with you here and us making breakfast together while it's snowing outside, I think this is the best Christmas ever."

"I do, too," she said, smiling back at him. Nothing else needed to be spoken. This was the best Christmas ever, and not one present had even been opened.

We were incredibly humbled at the outpouring of love and support for our family. I was grateful for the knowledge that my children would not remember this as the Christmas Lexi got diagnosed. Rather, it would be the Christmas we wanted more than anything to be together, the Christmas that everything was just as it had always been. This was only possible because so many took the time out of their lives to help care for our little family in our time of need.

Throughout the coming days, I thought a lot about charity. The world defines charity as "the voluntary giving of help, typically in the form of money, to those in need." Over the course of the last several months, we had found ourselves on the receiving end of so much support, presenting itself in so many different forms. It was never easy to be on the receiving end, especially in a situation like this, where we literally had nothing to give in return—not even our time. All we had and all we were was completely invested in our family, yet the love and kindness of others continued. Time and time again we found ourselves metaphorically and often literally in the embrace of friends and loved ones. I can understand the definition of charity that the world gives, but in our situation, it did not feel accurate.

We were being supported and strengthened in many ways, each one vital to us. Often I found myself wondering why. Why were we so fortunate to be encompassed by such wonderful and compassionate people? People who have put aside struggles in their own lives simply to try to lighten the load that our family was striving to bear. A second source—one that I hold to be far more accurate—states that charity is "the highest, noblest, strongest kind of love . . . even the pure love of Christ" (*Bible Dictionary*, "Charity"). Love is the key. It is what is missing in the first definition. We were not being surrounded or supported by someone looking for a tax write-off. We were being shown love—pure love. With every meal that had been prepared, every card or message sent, every visit, every prayer that had been uttered in our behalf, the world was being shown the true meaning of charity, and our family was eternally grateful for it. The unbearable became bearable.

The holidays had passed, and we were still soaring from the opportunity we had to spend them under the same roof. The time had come for Lexi to go back to the hospital for her fifth round of chemo. It was so nice to have an agenda of when we would be in the hospital and when we would be home, but cancer doesn't like to follow a schedule. Lab results showed that Lexi's platelets were too low for her to receive chemo that day. The doctors made the decision to postpone treatment for a week, hoping that she would recover herself.

She had come in for a transfusion (now a common occurrence) the previous Monday, and her ANC had continued to increase, which was a good sign, but her platelets had dropped again after the transfusion and hadn't gotten back up to where they were the day of transfusion. So we were sent home. While this sounds like a good thing—who wouldn't want to be at home instead of being in the hospital?—it is actually hard to hear that your child is not healthy enough for the life-saving treatment that she needs. When you are running a marathon, you don't want to stop for lunch in the middle. You want to continue on until you reach the end and then relax knowing that you can have a break at last.

A week filled with love and laughter passed. Again, we went into the clinic in hopes of seeing a sign that her body was recovering. Again, we were told that her body was not recovering as well as it should and her chemo could not yet be administered safely. Her doctors decided to give her body another week to make a comeback. The question was posed why Lexi wasn't just given more transfusions to boost her counts so that treatment could continue. The answer was quite simple: The body is a tricky thing and can become reliant on what it knows it is going to get. When transfusions are given too often, the body quits working so hard to recover itself, instead relying on a transfusion to rescue it. Thus, transfusions are given only when absolutely necessary. Over the course of treatment, Lexi would have over 130 medically necessary transfusions to sustain her body.

Another week passed only to reveal that Lexi was not yet healthy enough for chemo—again. We never thought we would be earnestly praying that she could get chemo, but we found ourselves doing just that. If she was healthy enough for chemo, it meant we could proceed with treatment, and even more than that, it meant her body was still able to recover itself from these horrific treatments. That was not the case this week. The following day we would head up to the hospital for yet another blood transfusion and then wait in hopes she would soon be well enough to proceed with treatment.

After being delayed for almost four weeks, the decision was made to begin chemo. Her body was still not recovering enough to reach the levels they deemed safe to continue, but they felt that her cancer could not go untreated any longer. It was a little bittersweet. For the past several weeks, we had been told repeatedly that it was unsafe for Lexi to continue chemo until her counts (blood, platelets, etc.) had reached a certain level. We were now being told that despite her counts not meeting those requirements, she needed to continue with treatment.

"We feel it has been too long," the doctors said, "and we are worried that if we continue to wait any longer, we might lose the ground we have gained. Her cancer is too aggressive to continue postponing. We will be monitoring her closely during recovery, and it is likely that she will need more transfusions than usual. Her body is just not recovering the way that we had anticipated."

My heart dropped. I wanted to proceed with treatment, not because I was antsy to go back to the hospital, or even because it meant moving forward. I wanted the confirmation that Lexi's body was still fighting back, that after this she would have the strength to return to her healthy self again. Their words did not give me the hope I so desperately needed at that time. Instead, I now had biological evidence that her body was struggling, and we were still in only the first step of treatment.

After her body recovered from this round, she would be going in for what the team referred to as a highly invasive surgery. Neuroblastoma likes to wrap itself around things. Due to the size and location of Lexi's tumor, it was surrounding many of her vital organs. We were told that the surgeon would remove as much of the tumor as was safely possible. Following surgery she still had another round of chemo, two stem cell transplants, radiation, antibody therapy, and then oral chemo. "This is our proposed road map for Lexi," the doctors said. "If we can get her through this, we will then re-evaluate to see how to proceed." Again, no guarantees.

I asked Lex if it bothered her when treatment or the undesirable nature of her tumor was discussed. She simply said, "Nope, I am not scared of the outcome. I know I will be fine. The journey is a little scary though."

This is where faith came in. My faith was not perfect. It did not yet replace all of my fears, but it had begun to outweigh them. Neil L. Andersen once said, "The future of your faith is not by chance, but by choice." We knew all too well that we would never know what events the future would hold for our family, cancer related or otherwise, but we did not need to know. We needed to focus on the things we had a choice in. We could choose to have faith and be strengthened by the peace that accompanied that choice.

Chapter Fourteen

I Am a God of Miracles

(2 Nephi 27:23)

*O*ur fifth round of chemo had officially ended, and we were learning how to navigate a little better between our two worlds. The cancer world can be all-consuming, but we felt strongly that life needed to progress outside of cancer as well, in hopes that life after cancer would not be as big of a transition. Observations had taught me that while a person—particularly a child—is battling cancer, they are put on somewhat of a pedestal. They are constantly praised, catered to, and receive copious amounts of attention and support, all rightfully so. Cancer is a monster that takes so much, so people often do anything and everything to offset the imbalance. The struggle in transition begins when a survivor no longer sports his or her bald head. The survivor has to begin learning to function in a world that isn't always quick to give praise or make exception.

As much as we wanted to give Lexi everything, we had to think about life after cancer. This meant that when we were at home, Lexi was still the big sister with all of the rights and responsibilities—modified, of course. She got to hang out with her friends and even had chores—greatly modified, but we still referred to them as chores. Mundane things like this helped her maintain a sense of life outside of cancer. She remembered life before and looked forward to life after.

That being said, she was not one to pass on an opportunity to laugh about the world she currently spent most of her time in. She decided to study for and take her driver's license permit test. She would be turning sixteen in eight months and wanted to begin practicing to get her license. We chose to stop at the Driver License Division on our way to the hospital one Monday morning. Lex and I walked in and found the permit applications. She began talking aloud as she filled out the paper work.

"Name: Alexis Michelle Gould. Height: 5'7". Weight: 105 pounds. Eye color: blue. Hair color . . ." She looked at me, and I just smiled as a small giggle escaped my mouth and I shrugged my shoulders. "Hair color: . . . nude!" She said in a voice loud enough to get a few stares. She laughed and took her paper to the desk, where they had her change her official hair color to brown. "Well," she said with a grin, "you can't blame a girl for trying."

Sometimes it felt as if it was just yesterday that Lexi had been diagnosed, and other days I struggled remembering life before cancer. One thing was certain though: time was passing. Cameron's appearance was evidence enough of that. When Lexi was diagnosed, Cam was shorter than I was. These days I found myself looking up to him, and I couldn't help but notice the thin brown line above his lip that was threatening to be facial hair. Livi was beginning to look less and less like a little girl and more like a young woman, and Aleah, not to be outdone, had begun to discover her own sense of style.

Surgery was next on the road map, and the day had come for our consultation with the surgeon. Lexi's surgery was scheduled for February 11. "Is there any chance that we could postpone the surgery for just a week?" Lexi asked the surgeon hopefully. "I don't usually like postponing treatment, but there is a sweethearts dance at my school. I'm not old enough to date yet, but a big group of my friends are going to go together. I was really hoping maybe I could go with them."

"I wish we could," he replied, "but your surgery is going to be very involved. I won't be able to do it alone, so I've asked two of my partners to clear their schedules for that day. The operating room has been blocked out for ten hours. Many accommodations needed to be made, and there isn't a way to change them back. I'm really sorry, Lexi."

"It's okay," she said with a small smile. "I understand. I didn't think so, but I just thought I'd ask."

The surgeon pulled up the scans taken earlier that week. Once again, the tumor was displayed in black and white before my eyes. As much as I wanted to look away, I couldn't. He went through the MRI images slide by slide to show us exactly how entwined this monstrosity had become with my daughter's organs. It encased major arteries and vessels. It displaced organs. It was the most prominent image on the screen. My teeth hurt from how hard I was clenching my jaw to keep it from quivering. My stomach turned, and I could feel myself becoming physically ill.

"The risk is that there isn't anything that this tumor is not affecting right now. The arteries it is encompassing are those that supply blood to the small intestine and the liver. As you know, she cannot live without either of these. Obviously we will do our best at avoiding damage to those, but arteries and vessels are fragile and can sustain damage by being disrupted in any way." He paused, giving us all a moment to grasp the situation.

"Neuroblastoma grows in clusters, and her tumor has grown so big so fast that it is completely encasing the aorta, as well as the major arteries that supply blood to the kidney, liver, pancreas, and spleen. We need to remove the tumor in its entirety for the best chance at remission, but we can't get too close to these arteries. Like I said, they don't like to be disrupted at all, let alone touched, and we are going to try to remove something that has grown completely around them."

The surgeon turned from the screen and asked Lexi to raise her shirt about six inches. With his pen he drew a line from each one of her ribs that angled slightly down, ending a few inches from her belly button. Another mock incision was made from there to just below her belly button, forming what resembled a *Y*. "This is the cut I plan on using. I've used it in the past and am comfortable with it. You'll have a pretty good scar after this, but I'll do my best to make it look as good as possible."

"I don't mind scars," Lexi replied with a smile. "I actually think they're cool!"

"Well," he said, "then you will be really impressed with my work in about a month!"

"About how much do you think you will be able to remove?" I mustered the courage to ask. I wanted a number to hold on to.

He blinked deliberately as he tried to find the words that were both realistic but factual. "We will do the best we can to remove as much of the tumor as possible. We may have to sacrifice a kidney, the spleen, and a portion of the liver or pancreas so that more of the tumor can be removed. But if that's what we need to do, we will do it. You can live without those things, and we need to remove as much of this as we can."

He continued with the risks of the procedure and what the plans were to offset them. In addition to the use of her port, she would need arterial lines in case of emergent transfusions. She would be intubated (placed on a machine that would breathe for her) during the entire surgery. She would spend some time in the Intensive Care Unit to recover following the surgery. Exactly how much time she would spend there would depend on her body. We left the consultation with confidence in our surgeon but not much else.

The next few weeks passed too quickly, as was the norm for any time at home. I tried to occupy my thoughts with the mundane, but my attempts in ignoring the words of the surgeon were futile. During the days, I found things to keep myself busy, but when I closed my eyes at night, I could see in grave detail my daughter's body on the operating table. Sleep once again eluded me. Kris seemed to be processing this next step in treatment better than I was.

"How are you so calm with what is coming up? I can't even close my eyes without wanting to scream. Why couldn't he give us a percentage? Even fifty percent—anything! You should've seen his eyes when he was talking with us. . . . That thing is wrapped around everything she needs in order to live. . . . Even if he's careful, it could be bad. . . . He kept saying how invasive it would be. . . ." I rambled on and on.

Kris turned to me with a vulnerability I had never before seen. As he spoke, his tear-filled eyes reflected a father's pure love. "I have to trust what we've been promised. I have put everything I am and all the energy I have into the promise that Heavenly Father has given us. I can't think about the alternative, because I won't survive it." Again, I was reminded that faith was not a product of strength but of trust. He had strength to do nothing but trust. We had strength to do nothing but trust.

While we were focusing on not focusing on the impending surgery, our friends had been focusing on making sure that Lexi did not miss her sweethearts dance after all. Several parents of the girls on Lexi's drill team decided that since she had already missed homecoming because of cancer, they could not let her miss sweethearts as well. They worked with her coaches and secured the dance room at the high school. I was told about their plans, and a few days before her surgery, Lexi and I went dress shopping. We came home from finding the perfect little black dress to a poster board and balloons on our front porch. Lexi had officially been asked to her first high school dance by the student body officers at her school.

Word had been sent out to friends and classmates. Practices from athletic teams were dismissed early, and kids dressed up to come to Lexi's sweethearts dance. A small table displayed a poster that read, "Love notes for Lexi." There were paper and pens for friends to write her encouraging messages. A backdrop had been set up for pictures, and a photographer had volunteered her time to photograph the kids.

As we were driving home that night, a genuine smile lit Lexi's face. Her eyes sparkled as she recounted the songs, the dances, and the friends that had worked so hard to give her this special gift. "Mom, this was probably the most fun night I have ever had." We all went to bed with smiles on our faces that night.

It was now the day before surgery, less than twenty-four hours before the time we would watch our daughter walk into surgery, not knowing where our path would lead. We had asked our bishop to come and give Lexi a blessing. Blessings had been accompanied by so much peace and comfort throughout this journey, and we knew we would need both to see us through. For some reason, I felt more anxious for her to get this blessing. My heart needed to hear the words that had been spoken to her before. I needed the confirmation that after everything that we had been told by medical professionals, the eternal promises that she had been given were still in effect. I needed to hear that Heavenly Father was still watching over her and that she really would be okay.

Our bishop and his wife came to our home, and we greeted them warmly. My heartbeat had been irregular for days now, and the pulsing in my chest had increased to the point of painful. I focused my breathing, and peace washed over me as our bishop told us that he had been fasting for two days and had just come from the temple. He wanted to be certain that the words he was about to say were indeed the words Heavenly Father would have him speak. My heart knew that this blessing would hold the fate of our daughter. I prayed earnestly that it was still the same as what had been promised in the prior months.

The blessing began, and my world stopped turning. I was determined to hear every word spoken, process every sentence uttered, and understand every blessing promised. Again we were reminded as in times before that this was not the end of Lexi's mortal journey but a preparation for things she would accomplish in this life. But this blessing was more in depth than the others. We were told that Lexi was not alone in this fight, that she literally had an army behind her—one that she could see and one that she could not. My eyes filled as I felt the presence of more than just the physical bodies in the room. The blessing continued, and Lexi was told that she would see miracles. That God would show others, through her, that the power of the priesthood was real and miracles still happened on the earth.

My entire life I had read stories in the scriptures about the miracles of God. I often thought of how it would be to behold the miracle of the loaves and fishes, or be the mother of a stripling warrior who had returned after battle. I thought of watching my children wait patiently for their turn to be held and blessed by Jesus Christ. I was being told that I would witness a modern-day miracle, something so beautiful that nothing short of the word "miracle" would suffice. I no longer felt any frustration for what my daughter would go through. Humbleness permeated my heart as I came to know that Heavenly Father would allow His works to be manifest through our trials. Sadness and pain were still constant companions, but they were based on what she would feel, not why she would feel it.

Sometimes we expect that if we are truly living the gospel, we will feel nothing but happiness all the time. This is not the case. If we were never meant to feel other emotions, why did Heavenly Father send us with them? Even innocent children can feel sadness. Christ felt sad. It is okay if we do. The difference is that even in our most extreme times of sadness and heartache, an underlying calmness can accompany our troubled hearts. We can be filled with a sense of understanding and comfort in knowing that we will overcome even the most unbearable of circumstances. The blessing concluded, and the feeling of peace in our home was tangible. Embraces were given amidst the watering of every eye in the room.

We thanked the bishop and his wife for their time and the experience we had just shared. No sooner did we see them out and sit on our couch than our doorbell rang. I opened the door to unexpectedly find my sister and her family on my front porch. Behind them stood our entire family. Brothers, sisters, grandmas, nieces, and nephews were all standing on our front porch and onto the lawn. My heart felt as if it would burst as they filed in one by one, hugging me as they passed. They sat down and my sister looked to me.

"We just knew you guys were nervous about tomorrow." Our eyes filled with tears in unison as the big sister that used to let me tag along on her adventures could feel the pain that my mom heart was trying to disguise. "It didn't seem enough to just call and tell you we love you over the phone. We just thought you could all use a big group hug." At that moment, each of them rose and literally circled us in the arms of their love. We simultaneously laughed at the size of the group hug (it numbered more than thirty souls) and cried together.

The excitement and emotion from the group hug had not fully subsided when our doorbell rang again. We opened it to find all of the young women in our ward and their leaders. The Young Women president spoke. "We just came by to sing to you and let you know how much we love you. We will all be praying for you tomorrow." Any hope of getting my watery eyes under control was quickly abandoned as they sang. The Spirit with which they bore testimony through song filled every nook, cranny, and heart in our home.

We slept that night and woke early in the morning to have a family prayer and head to the hospital. I was surprised to learn that there was an express lane when it came to surgery check-in. We were rushed from one room to the next. Instructions were reiterated in an abbreviated version and papers were signed saying that we understood the risks accompanying the procedure.

The anesthesiologist entered the room and told us how he would put Lexi to sleep and keep her sedated throughout the surgery. "She will need to be heavily sedated due to the nature and length of the surgery. When the body is as heavily sedated as hers will be, it forgets to breathe on its own, so she will be intubated. This just means that she will have a tube going down her throat that is hooked up to a machine that will breathe for her." I focused on remembering to breathe myself as vivid horrors flooded my mind once again. He continued, "I am not as concerned with during the surgery as I am with after the surgery. Pain control will be a big issue. The organs and intestines do not like to be bothered. The doctors will be greatly disrupting all of them. In addition to that, her incision will be quite large and very deep. They will be cutting through the muscles in the abdomen in order to get to the tumor. These are core muscles in the abdomen that are used for almost any type of movement. Recovery will be brutal."

While I appreciated his honesty, I think I could have stood a little less detail. I thought he was done, but he began again. "She is going to be coming out of surgery with multiple drains and tubes, one of which is a chest tube. This will help any excess fluid drain from her lungs and chest cavity. They are extremely painful, as they sit right between the ribs. I need to place an epidural to help offset this pain." We nodded our understanding.

Again he continued, but in a more subdued tone. "An epidural is placed into one of many small epidural veins in the back. Many times during the placement, one of the veins is nicked without us knowing because they are so small. This is generally not a concern, because the body can easily and quickly stop the bleeding making it a safe procedure . . . usually. That is not the case for Lexi. As you are aware, normal platelet counts can range anywhere from 150–450 thousand. In order to do this surgery safely, we wanted her platelets to be at least seventy-five thousand. They were at sixty-two thousand today. The surgery cannot be postponed. They transfused, hoping to get her platelets higher, but they couldn't. If an epidural vein in Lexi's body were to get nicked without us knowing, she would bleed to death. The risk is far too great. I cannot safely place the epidural. She greatly needs it, but I cannot place it." He apologized again and said he would do everything he could to minimize the pain but reiterated that her body was limiting what could be done. She would have to endure more pain than we had thought.

The anesthesiologist left us with each other and our thoughts as he exited the room. A surgical nurse came in, and before I knew it, we were saying good-bye to our daughter. We kissed her head and kissed her again.

"Love you guys," she said with a soft smile. "I'll see you soon."

"Love you, baby girl," we said, and then we watched her stand a little taller as she squared her shoulders and walked down the hall with her nurse.

We hadn't fully rounded the corner before I crumbled into Kris's arms. He held me as I quietly sobbed. A few minutes passed, and I collected myself enough to face our family in the waiting room. Grandmas, aunts, uncles, and Lexi's drill team coaches all came to wait with us for what proved to be one of the longest days of our lives. Hand in hand, Kris and I greeted them and found a place to sit. They had brought food and games to help pass the time, but all I could do was wait for the hourly phone call we had been promised to keep us updated on the progress of the surgery.

About thirty minutes had passed from the time Lexi had left our side when her surgeon approached us in the waiting room. We were caught off guard to see him wearing a button-up shirt, slacks, and a tie. I had never been to medical school, but I was fairly certain that this was not typical surgical attire. "Lexi is doing well. They have put her breathing tube in and started the general anesthetic. Her arterial lines have been placed, and all of her vitals are being monitored. I apologize. I was hoping to get to speak with her before she went back, but I didn't make it in time."

He continued, "There is a renowned surgeon visiting from New York, and he was holding grand rounds this morning. His specialty is the removal of neuroblastoma tumors. I attended the rounds in which he emphasized the importance of the removal of the tumor in its entirety and introduced an alternative incision that I would like to use on Lexi." He used his pen to indicate the path in the air in which he would cut into our daughter's body. "Rather than make two small incisions that join in the Y shape as I was planning on before, I would like to start farther back on the left side and have it curve down past her belly button. It is a larger incision that will cut directly through her diaphragm, which will make for a more painful recovery, but I believe it will give us greater access to the tumor."

A feeling of peace washed over me. It was not enough to absolve all of my fears, but it was enough to help me recognize the tender mercy of a leading renowned surgeon being present on the very day our daughter was being operated on. Confirmation came, and once again, I could feel that Lexi was being watched over and protected.

Our first update came an hour and forty minutes after Lexi had left our side. In addition to her port being accessed, the anesthesiologist had to place a central line in her neck to monitor the blood flow in her heart, an arterial line to monitor blood pressure with each heart beat, and a few IVs that would allow for large quantities of blood to be transfused in a short amount of time. All of the prep had just finished, and the incision had been made.

The nurse asked if I had any questions. I said no and thanked her for the update. "Um, Mrs. Gould," she said, "I was talking to Lexi right before she fell asleep, and she was really concerned about you and her dad. She said she knew you would be worrying about her all day. I told her I would be the one calling and updating you." Her voice caught slightly. "Lexi asked that every time I call to give you an update, I tell you that she loves you very much. She said you would need to hear it."

My lip trembled as I pictured our fifteen-year-old daughter lying on the operating table. So many things could have been running through her head—and yet she expressed concern for our well-being. I tried to steady my voice and replied softly, "I know she is already asleep and can't hear, but will you please whisper in her ear that her mom and dad love her very much?" The nurse agreed, and I thanked her with a mother's tearful heart. My soul filled with gratitude as I realized that even though we could not physically be by Lexi's side during this process, we were not far from her heart or her from ours.

I now looked forward to the phone calls, not only for the update, but also for how they ended every time—"Mrs. Gould, Lexi wants you to know that she loves you and her dad very much."

"Please tell her we love her very much too," I would always say.

As the day continued on, my mind felt the weight of our situation. It was as if I had run an emotional marathon in quicksand. Every phone call said the same thing: "They are still working on removing the tumor . . . Remember that Lexi loves you." Until the last call came.

"This is Emily Gould," I said. I was surprised when a man's voice responded. It was the surgeon instead of his nurse on the line.

"Surgery went well—actually, the best it could've gone. As you know, her tumor was centrally located and was encasing many major arteries and vessels." I paused for our moment of truth, bracing myself to learn what organs had to be lost in order to give us the best chance of winning this fight. I wondered how much more still lurked inside her. He continued. "We were able to remove the tumor entirely."

My voice caught, and tears filled my eyes and began to spill over. "I'm sorry, you said that her tumor was completely removed? All of it? What organs needed to be sacrificed?"

He patiently waited until my flood of questions had come to an end. "Yes, we removed all of it, everything that we could see. There is no more visible neuroblastoma in Lexi's abdomen. Also, she was able to keep all of her organs. We did not need to take any of them. They all look to be healthy and functioning."

I gathered myself enough to thank him with everything I had and hung up the phone. The same man who told us our daughter had cancer had just told me that he had been able to remove her entire tumor piece by piece.

I turned into Kris's waiting arms and sobbed. "It's gone, they got it all out. He removed all of the tumor, and she has all of her organs—everything. It is truly a miracle." I continued to sob. "It's gone, all of it. It's really gone," I whispered, not fully believing what was coming out of my mouth. Our family (her drill coaches had long since been considered family) embraced us and one another as I held tight to Kris. Ten minutes after our first call, we received a second one.

"Hello Mrs. Gould, this is the anesthesiologist. We just did a post-op platelet count on Lexi. Her platelets are over two hundred thousand, and I can safely place the epidural that she needs, if that is okay with you." My mind was still reeling from our previous news. I couldn't believe what I was hearing and assumed it must be a mistake. Her platelets had not reached more than seventy-five since her first round of chemo.

"I'm sorry, are you sure? We are talking about Alexis Gould, right?" I asked.

"Yes," he replied. "I had them check it twice because I did not believe it myself. I don't know how, but her platelets are over two hundred thousand now. I can place the epidural she needs without the fears I had before. It is completely safe and will save her from immense pain."

Again, we saw an unexplained miracle. Her platelets dropped just a day or two later. Throughout treatment, and for months after, they never again reached one hundred thousand.

Another hour passed as we waited for the okay to go see her. Finally, after being away from our daughter for more than twelve hours, Kris and I headed to the ICU, hand in hand, to see Lexi. She would need to spend the next few days there to make sure she was recovering well. We entered our daughter's small ICU room. There was no chatter as she was waking up from anesthetic this time, only a furrowed brow accompanied by the occasional moan or whimper.

Her entire body was swollen and sore. One of her arms had been wrapped to a board, and we were told this was to secure the arterial line. Several tubes were leading into and out of her petite frame. Because of the breathing tube that was still in place, it was extremely difficult for her to speak. We reached her side, and each of us held one of her hands in ours. Her eyes remained shut as she mustered all her strength to feebly squeeze our hands. We gently squeezed back, and her tired eyes tried to open. As we held her hands, we whispered to her that the tumor, in its entirety, was gone. Her lip began to quiver around the breathing tube, and she whispered, "It's a miracle. He promised I would see miracles, and this is a miracle."

Miracles happen every day all around us. Some we recognize as miracles, and some we write off as coincidence. I knew that what happened with Lexi was too much of a coincidence to be just a coincidence. I knew it was the priesthood blessings, along with the combined faith, prayers, fasting, thoughts, love, and support of so many that brought a modern-day miracle to pass. I vowed that regardless of what the future held, I would never forget the events of this day and the blessings we had witnessed. In no way could I have ever prepared myself for the way in which this promise would be tested in the coming months.

Chapter Fifteen

Remembering the Tender Mercies
(Psalm 25:6)

The following morning, the surgeon entered our ICU room, and in a hoarse whisper, Lexi asked, "Was it just a dream, or did you really remove all of my tumor?" His eyes glistened, and he confirmed that it was gone. He examined her and remarked that she was doing very well in spite of the extensiveness of her surgery. A few hours later, her oncologist stopped in to check on her. Despite Lexi's inability to physically move her own limbs, she bore witness to what she knew to be true. With great effort, Lexi asked, "Did you hear about my miracle?"

The oncologist shook her head slightly. Lexi then slowly told her about the removal of her tumor. The oncologist glanced at me with a puzzled look, wondering exactly how much pain medication Lexi had been given. She had seen the imaging and knew what we were up against. She looked at me, and I could do no more than nod in affirmation. The oncologist then looked back to Lexi and, with a tear on her cheek, confirmed that the removal of a tumor of that size and position was indeed a miracle. Satisfied, Lexi again closed her eyes and fell back asleep, completely worn out by the brief interaction.

Life in the ICU is like a day that never ends. The lights are never dimmed, and voices are never hushed. It is like living in a constant state of emergency and panic. After one night there, I understood why they said that weeks in the ICU can lead a person to fits of psychosis. A nurse is constantly stationed in your room, monitoring the patient, and while you are grateful for the diligence, it makes sleep unattainable. When your body decides to finally give in due to sheer exhaustion, a deafening alarm from either your room or someone else's is sure to sound, indicating a medical emergency. If it is from your room, any hope of sleep completely eludes you for hours on end. If not, you find yourself lying hopelessly on your reclining chair that doubles as your bed, your heart breaking for the parent whose child set off the alarm.

We were grateful to learn that after only two nights and a day, Lexi was stable enough to be transferred to her own room on the surgical unit to finish recovery. The surgeon thought she would need to stay inpatient only another seven to ten days for recovery before heading home. Her breathing tube was removed, making it so we only had to transport nine tubes and drains to our new living quarters. She was currently unable to lift her head or even turn it from side to side. She talked only when it was completely necessary, and with great effort. Her physical therapy started with her learning to wiggle the finger we pointed to and then graduated to her gaining enough strength to lift her arm.

We had only been in our room for thirty hours when we were visited by the surgical team, but this time the look on their faces told me that this visit was not merely to check on Lexi's progress in recovery. The surgeon pulled up an image on the screen. "The routine imaging that we've been doing to check for internal bleeding has revealed free air in her abdomen that has not been present in previous X-rays. This is an indication of a tear in Lexi's intestine. We need to take her in for a second surgery immediately in order to make sure that her intestines are intact and there is no damage. There is no other choice." He left, and the nurse came in shortly to prepare Lexi with her accompanying tubes and drains to go back down to the OR.

For the second time in three days, we watched as our daughter left us to head into surgery. There would be no squaring of the shoulders and walking alongside the nurse. This time her bed would be wheeled down a quiet hall while we silently watched it venture past doors we weren't allowed to go through. This time there was no busy waiting room, no games or distractions, no updates—just Kris and I sitting in an empty waiting room on a lonely Sunday night, once again waiting to hear that our daughter would be okay.

A few hours passed before the surgeon came out to speak to us. "I was very thorough. I went through section by section of her intestines." He motioned the action he had taken, and I decided that surgeons should keep their arms folded when talking to the parents of their patients. "Luckily I did not find any damage, and the intestines look completely intact." I exhaled loudly, grateful for the words he spoke. "However," he continued, "she will need to stay in the ICU again, probably for longer than before."

I looked at him quizzically. This surgery was far less invasive, and she had already been moved to the surgical recovery unit. I wondered why we couldn't just go back up to our room. He saw my questioning gaze and explained further. "The intestines and the internal organs do not like to be disturbed at all, and we've been very aggressive with them twice in three days. Her body was not well enough for one major surgery, and now she will have to find a way to recover from two." We were then led to Lexi's ICU room and found her the same way we had just a few days before. It was a horrible case of déjà vu that made my stomach turn. We reached Lexi's bedside to find that she was indeed more exhausted than she had been following her first surgery. There was no attempt made to squeeze our hands or open her eyes. Her breathing tube was firmly in place, and it was clear she did not have the energy to try to speak around it.

Kris made sure that we were both okay and then headed home to maintain balance for Cam, Liv, and Aleah. I tried to settle in the best that I could but found that the concept of time once again eluded me. The clock on the wall kept ticking, telling me that minutes, hours, and days were passing by, but it didn't register. It seemed that time dragged on and yet remained motionless. Lexi's vitals began to stabilize, and we transferred again to the surgical floor to recover. It was evident already that this time around, things would be more difficult. For several days following the second surgery, she lay immobile on her bed, trying not to move in an effort to minimize the pain. Even the small progress she had made following her first surgery appeared to have been lost. Her body had fought to take one step forward and had just been pushed ten steps back. My days and most nights that first week were spent on a chair next to her bed. Holding her hand seemed to bring her an unspoken comfort.

Slowly she began to be able to take a few short steps at a time. She was unstable at best and needed constant support. Her first few steps came at great expense. No words were spoken, just a grip on my arms as we inched our way a few feet. Her teeth chattered from the pain, and her body shook. We returned to her bed, and I helped lower her back into the only position her body tolerated. By this time, the pain had caused her heart rate to go well over two hundred.

"Lexi, what would you rate your pain right now?" her nurse asked.

"9.5," Lexi responded with much effort.

Her nurse shook her head and replied, "You are my hero, Lex. I can tell that on a scale of one to ten, your pain is at least a twelve, and you still won't say ten."

Lexi took a moment to compose herself before responding. "I'm saving my ten for when I have babies," she said through chattering teeth. I smiled sadly, thinking of the heartache that her statement could hold in the future.

"Sis, I have had four babies, and I can assure you that I have never gone through what you are going through. You can use your ten," I said, trying to lighten the pang in my heart.

She smiled weakly as she continued to shake, her body still trying to calm down. I watched helplessly and tried to control my voice in an effort to offer comfort. Finally, she was stabilized again, and I resumed my hand-holding responsibility, knowing that in a few short hours the process would need to be repeated.

Livi and Aleah were not yet allowed to visit, but Kris and Cam came often to check on Lexi and see her progress. She always saved her best walk of the day for her dad.

After four days of this excruciating process, I was helping Lexi walk. As she leaned heavily on me, she whispered, "Mama, I hurt so bad. How much longer before it starts getting better? I just hurt."

I silently prayed. How much more would she have to endure before the pain lessened? "I'm so sorry, my baby," I whispered in her ear as I strived to keep my voice from cracking. "I'm so, so sorry."

I felt her slightly lift her head to try to look in my eyes. "It's okay. My tumor is dead and I am not, so I still won." She had been beaten down, yet somehow she still showed fight. She could not yet move on her own accord, yet she was so much stronger than I was.

My weakened heart pleaded with my Father in Heaven as my daughter struggled to inch closer to her bed, her head leaning on my shoulder because it took too much energy to hold it upright. "Father," I silently spoke, "I know she will do everything you ask, and I am trying to, but I can't do this anymore. I can't watch helplessly without an end in sight. I know we've witnessed miracles, and I will forever be grateful to Thee for that, but I pray, please, Father, take some of this from her—for my sake. She is strong enough. I am not." I humbly closed my prayer as I helped lower Lexi back into her bed. I held her hand while her body calmed down from the exertion and then silently continued my plea as I wept at her bedside.

The following morning I woke to a soft "Hi, Mama." I turned to see Lex tiredly looking at me and slightly smiling.

"Hey, honey," I responded, grateful for a smile. "How are you feeling?"

"Tired, but a little better," she replied. There was a difference in her countenance and less difficulty when she spoke. She fell back asleep as a glimmer of hope entered my heart. She awoke a few hours later, and it was time for our walk. "I want to try to go outside of my room today," she said. "I'm still in a lot of pain, but I'm feeling a little stronger. Can we try to go to the nurse's desk outside?" I agreed, and we began the slow process of preparing her for a walk.

We opened the door to her room, and she continued slowly, inches at a time, to head to the nurse's desk, about ten feet from our door. She touched the desk only to ask if we could go farther still. I should've known. Lexi sets goals only to beat them. Carefully and methodically we continued on.

"There is actually a fart gun at the end of this hall," one of the nurses said. I saw an impish grin play across Lexi's lips and realized that she had set a new goal for herself. I looked in her clear eyes, and she nodded slightly. We then began the twenty-foot trek to the end of our hall.

The pain grew with every step, but so did her determination. She began to shake and hold tighter to my arms, her head resting on my shoulder. All of her focus would need to be on her goal if she was to attain it. Little by little we made our way to the end of the hall, pausing when the pain became unbearable. Her jaw clenched and her eyes watered, but she refused to let a single tear escape. I asked if she wanted to turn back, told her that she had far exceeded any walk up to this point and we could try again later, but she was adamant.

She would not quit until she had reached her goal. We had been walking for over fifteen minutes and had made it the thirty feet from the bed to the fart gun. She lifted it gingerly and looked at me as her penciled-in eyebrows went up. With a smile she pulled the trigger. She quietly giggled and then pulled it again. I laughed and wondered if anyone else was enjoying the fact that a fart gun was such a huge motivator for a fifteen-year-old girl.

"You've helped me realize something today, Lex," I said. "Dad and I are raising one classy lady!" Her smile broadened as she pulled the trigger one last time. Slowly, we began the trail back to her room.

The walk did not come without consequences, but a change had definitely taken place over the last twenty-four hours. All of the same signs and symptoms were present, but she had been made physically stronger to be able to bear them. I marveled at the change I saw, knowing it was the answer to the plea of a brokenhearted mother.

"Lex," I said once she was settled back in her bed, "you are the strongest person I know."

She contemplated this. "Mom, people say I'm strong, but I have never been so weak. I need help sitting, standing, and walking. I'm just barely getting the strength to lift my own head and arms again. I don't feel strong."

I gathered my thoughts before I responded. "Physical strength is an attribute that anyone can have and anyone can lose at any time, without any notice." She nodded in agreement, knowing all too well how true this was. "Your strength comes from your faith, your mind, your kindness, and your genuine love for others. Cancer, like many trials, works to reveal the character of a person—who you really are when things are at the lowest point. You are continually being tried, yet you continue to shine brighter. When it would be the easiest to become bitter, you strive to be better. There are many things that cancer can and will take from you. But it will never take who you are, and that is the most powerful type of strength a person can possess." She smiled at me sleepily and slowly drifted off to sleep, resting up for when Kris came to visit. She was excited to show him what was at the end of the hall.

It had been two weeks since Lexi's second surgery, and every day we saw minor improvements in some form. Whether it was that she was able to pull her chest tube out (she chose to do this in front of Cam in an effort to gross him out—it worked) or that she was able to eat a few bites of food. Progress was real and undeniable. The days were long and hard. We often took two steps forward and one step back, but as I looked over my shoulder at the past two weeks, I knew we were heading in the right direction.

Over the course of the previous weeks, I had seen my daughter suffer in a way that I did not know was physically possible. I watched her body writhe in pain, unable to do anything to make it stop. She had hit what I deemed to be a physical rock bottom, more than once. I was not sure that she could possibly endure anymore. However, amidst the heartache, we could not help but be reminded of the miracle that was ours. The suffering that she had gone through from the surgery would have been there if only a portion of the tumor had been removed, but it wasn't. The entire tumor was removed, all of it. We had seen a miracle, and we could not deny it. In the middle of the heart-wrenching recovery, I felt strength knowing that we had been blessed beyond what we thought possible.

Sometimes in life great things happen, and then hard times come, and we are quick to forget the blessings we have been given. I knew that this journey of ours was far from over. I knew that difficult times lay ahead, but I vowed to never forget the miracle we had beheld and the undeniable fulfillment of God's promise we had witnessed. I had been given the knowledge that the faith and prayers of many had brought that miracle to pass, and I was determined to spend my days with gratitude in my heart for this precious gift.

Chapter Sixteen

Thy Faith Hath Made Thee Whole
(Matthew 9:22)

*S*everal years ago, when Cam was a baby, he had to stay the night at Primary Children's Hospital because of respiratory problems. Once he was asleep, I ventured to the cafeteria and was feeling quite sorry for myself and my sick little boy. As I neared the cafeteria, I passed a mom pulling her beautifully bald-headed child in a wagon. She had a radiant smile on her face as she exclaimed, "Look, sweetheart, we get to go outside of your room today!" Her genuine happiness, despite her circumstance, caused me to reset my thinking. I vowed that day to never again have pity for the circumstances I found myself in and to forever be grateful for the health of my children.

Life often comes full circle on us. It was an unusually warm February afternoon, and for the first time in over two weeks, Lexi was able to go outside. As I was pushing her wheelchair, she looked up at me with a radiant smile and said, "Mom, I can't believe we get to go outside today!" My mind was transported back to that mother, and I was reminded of the humility I felt so long ago, of silently praying for forgiveness for focusing on my menial trials, and of the promise I had made to forever be grateful. I never spoke to that mother. She would never know the impact she had on me. But that day, as I pushed my beautiful bald-headed baby outside, I was reminded of the lessons she taught me so many years ago.

Just over three weeks had passed, and we finally had a discharge date. We left on a Sunday and then returned for our next round of chemo on Wednesday.

Our sixty-four hours of home time was up, and we headed to the hospital for what was to be our last round of chemo. Lexi was hooked up, and the medication was pumped into her veins. I was unprepared for the emotions that flooded my mind. I should be happy—elated, even. This was her last round of chemo. The happiness came but was overpowered by other emotions. Step one would be officially completed with this round of chemo. Step two had been completed upon discharge from surgery. In my mind, I knew that this meant that step three was up next—transplant. Fears and emotions that had been stored in the recesses of my mind now came to the forefront. New worries and old conversations regarding transplant replayed in my head like a horrible movie that grew more intense when I closed my eyes.

"Mom, have you had lunch yet?" Lexi's voice broke through my thoughts.

"Not yet, but I will."

"Mom, it's time for lunch, and I don't want you to forget to eat."

Somehow she had found out that I had a habit of forgetting to regularly eat when she was inpatient. This was a side effect that I didn't even realize was happening until someone pointed it out. I had always had such a healthy appetite, putting many teenage boys to shame. But there was something about being inpatient and seeing what Lex had to go through that caused my appetite to be nonexistent. Over the past few months, Lexi had made it her mission to make sure I ate regularly, even asking the nurses to remind me if she knew she would be unable to because of her meds. I smiled at the thought of her being concerned about me when she was the patient, and I decided I could use a walk anyway.

Parts of PCMC were still under construction from when Lex first started treatment. I never tired of walking past the drawings and words of encouragement written by patients and loved ones on the temporary sheetrock. As I was walking to the cafeteria, I passed a piece of sheetrock that Lexi had written on during a previous visit. In her handwriting I read the words of what had been the first scripture she had ever memorized. "I will not leave you comfortless. I will come to you" (John 14:18). This particular scripture had always been her favorite, but it had come to offer new meaning over the last few months.

During this time when I was struggling to find peace and comfort, I resolved to hold to these words as if they were my lifeline, because on some days they quite literally were. I could choose to focus on my fears, or I could choose to find comfort in someone much greater than myself. I could choose to feel isolated and alone, like no one could possibly understand the heartache that we were enduring. Or I could choose to realize that not only did someone understand perfectly what I was going through, but He also understood what Kris was going through. He had suffered through Lexi's pain and Cameron's heartache. He felt Olivia's fears and Aleah's worries. And He did all of this willingly, so that He would have the ability to perfectly succor us in our time of need. I did not know what was to come. Who really does know everything that life will hold? But I knew that my energy was much more wisely spent focusing on the things that I could accomplish today rather than fretting about the fears of tomorrow.

The following days held no surprises, and we were home together within a week. Transplant was quickly approaching, so we decided to make the most of the limited time that we had been given. Each year, the Spinnakers held a year-end review, in which they showcased each of their dances. Although she had two major surgeries just a few weeks prior, Lexi was determined to dance. Her coaches and teammates worked with her patiently, and the dance that had been performed for her just a few months before was modified so that she could perform it with her team.

The night of review had come, and for the first time since that fateful September afternoon, Lexi put glitter on her eyelids and applied her red lipstick. She put on her gold spankies and the shirt that bore her name. She worked so hard to look like every other member of her drill team, but more than just her bald head gave away the fact that she was different. That night she danced as if she didn't know when or if she would dance again—because she didn't. She had learned that what most kids take for granted—getting up early to go to school or practice, being able to do chores or hold a job, having the chance to be at home—should never be taken lightly. They were gifts, opportunities. She was now determined to forever see the mundane as a blessing.

The following weeks were filled with numerous appointments. Every inch of Lexi was poked, prodded, scanned, and tested. At last, the final day of appointments and scans had arrived. We were checked in and led back to a private room. "Someone has good taste in music," Lexi said as she walked into our room.

"That's Ricky," the tech replied. "You've met him, haven't you?"

Lexi replied with a shake of her head, and the tech knocked on the door across the hall from ours. She opened it and stuck her head in, likely asking if the occupants were up for the interaction. Without warning, a six-foot, two-inch, seventeen-year-old boy came out into the hall with a full head of dark brown hair and a bright smile. "Hey! I'm Ricky," he said warmly.

Clearly taken back by the fact that he was not only a teenager but also a teenager with hair, Lex took half a second to respond. "Hey, I'm Lexi," she said with a smile. "We were just eavesdropping on your music."

"Aw, ya like that?" he replied. "I'm a big fan of Drake—well, that and making my mama laugh, and she's always laughing when I try to dance." Ricky then showcased what he believed were his best dance moves amid the laughter of Lexi, his mom, and the nurses. Too soon a dietician came, reminding us what we were actually there for, and we said our good-byes to our new friends.

The dietician went over what foods transplant patients were allowed to safely eat—things like cantaloupe and any type of berries didn't make the cut. Any fresh fruit or vegetables that she wished to eat would need to be washed thoroughly with soap and water, rinsed, and then washed again. Any utensils or dishes used to prepare her food would need to go through the same process. All meat would need to be thoroughly cooked (a big blow, considering Lexi's favorite meal was rare steak), and she would not be able to use the same jar of peanut butter, container of sour cream, or bag of chips as anyone else. She would be on what they referred to as a low-microbial diet. Lexi referred to it as "the not being able to eat anything that was actually good" diet.

Next, the pharmacist entered and went over the plethora of medications that Lexi would receive, in hopes of minimizing the effects of the high-dose chemo and the transplant. I thought that her med list was long before, but I soon realized that there are multiple medications that they reserve for transplant patients only. I think I could have happily gone through my life without having the knowledge of these drugs, why she would need them, and what the side effects of minimizing other side effects could possibly be.

After the scanning, testing, and visits from the dietician and pharmacist, our social worker entered the room. We had grown quite fond of her over the previous months, and we greeted each other warmly. "Well," she began, "I am actually here for professional reasons." She looked at Lexi and then me and uncomfortably went on. "So, my job with transplant patients is to make sure that they have taken the time to let their family members know their wishes." I was taken aback. Surely I had misheard her.

"Lexi, do you understand what she is saying?" I asked, praying my voice held steady. Lexi shook her head slightly. Our social worker rushed on, apologetically, knowing the words she had to speak but not loving the fact they had to be spoken.

"The chemo you will be given is potentially fatal, Lexi. In the case that this transplant does not take and your body cannot be rescued, we have found that it is much easier for the family and those left behind to make a decision when it has been discussed beforehand. The family will have an easier time letting go if they know that's what the patient wants." She stopped and looked at Lexi, who still did not show that she fully comprehended what was being said.

"Exactly what do you mean?" Lexi asked. It wasn't that she didn't grasp what was being said; it was simply that the idea that she might not survive had never occurred to her.

I looked at her carefully. "Lex, honey, they want you to have a talk with dad and I to let us know how long you would like to be on life support if the transplant does not take. They want us to talk about how long you would like your life sustained before we let you pass." The words felt sick in my mouth and left a horrible taste that no amount of swallowing would get rid of.

Oddly enough, it was not just the physical loss of our child that haunted me. That thought alone could not be fathomed, but it was more than that. It was knowing that we would have to stand idly by, completely helpless, and watch her endure the unspeakable. We would have to watch her body come so close to death and not be able to do anything to stop it. We knew it was coming, and we would have to sign papers saying that we would be "okay" with it. Could any parent ever truly be okay with this?

With a lightness in her tone that didn't match the weight of the conversation, Lexi replied, "Oh, okay. Well, I don't want to live on machines at all. If it's my time to go, then I'll go. Just let me go."

Surprised by her honest yet simple answer, I quickly said, "Well honey, it is something that we would prayerfully discuss. I don't think it is that simple."

Our social worker piped up. "Your mom is right. It is quite an emotional and thoughtful process. I hate even bringing it up, but it is part of my job with transplant patients."

"It's okay," Lexi replied. "I was promised that I will be fine, so I'm not worried. The transplant will take, and I will make it through."

Her faith was contagious, and I found myself once again rejuvenated by her confidence in the sacred promises she had been given. We thanked our social worker and awaited the arrival of the doctors who were going to review the results of Lexi's scans with us. I reminded myself that breathing was still a mandatory thing and concentrated on the rising and falling of my chest as the longest five minutes of my life passed. They entered the room and began pulling up images of the inside of my daughter on the screen. They silently read the report and then turned to us. I met their gaze, and my world stopped.

"Well," they began, "the results of Lexi's scans are back, and all of them show no evidence of disease."

I leaned a little closer, not sure if my ears had actually heard these results or if my heart had dreamt them up. "I'm sorry, what did you say?"

"Lexi's scans came back clear. There is no evidence of disease in her body."

I clenched my jaw to keep it from trembling and willed my eyes to not well with tears. Both attempts proved to be futile. They must have seen this reaction often because they continued on as normal. "This means that although there are still likely cancer cells in her body, they are small enough that the tests and scans cannot detect any."

I felt as if confetti should be falling from the ceiling and a giant jumbotron should drop displaying Lexi's face with the words "NO EVIDENCE OF DISEASE!" written on the bottom of the screen. It doesn't quite happen like that, but I couldn't have been more excited if it would have.

This amazing news did not alter Lexi's treatment plan at all. Although nothing was visible on a scan, years of research has shown that in order to have the best chance of staying in remission, each step of a patient's road map must be completed. She was scheduled to be admitted for her first stem-cell transplant on April 12. We would likely stay inpatient for about four weeks, come home for a week, and then be admitted for another four weeks for her second transplant. After that, she would need radiation, followed by six months of antibody therapy. We still had a long road ahead of us, but we were on the right path. The doctors continued on with the rest of the testing results.

The remainder of the results weren't as positive as we had hoped; however, given the news we had just received, I couldn't help but maintain a slight smile. I doubt anything could have dampened my mood right then. As it turned out, the chemotherapy Lexi had been on had caused significant hearing loss in high-frequency tones. Luckily, most speech sounds are made in the lower frequencies, so this result was not expected to have a huge impact on her ability to communicate with others. The decision was made that at that point she did not need a hearing aid. They would just closely monitor her hearing throughout the rest of treatment. She had also sustained a moderate to severe defect in her pulmonary (lung) function. This would not make it difficult for her to breathe, but it would affect her lung capacity.

Cancer takes you from tears of joy to tears of sorrow in a matter of minutes. Although I had begun to master my leaky eyes a little better over the past few months, I still struggled hearing the damage that had already occurred in Lexi's body and knowing that we hadn't even gotten to the most difficult part of treatment yet. As the lasting price she would pay for survival was explained to us, I felt an odd sense of peace and comfort. I was profoundly grateful for the blessings Lexi had received that promised her the opportunity to fully and completely return to everything she loved doing. Being reminded of those blessings gave me strength to hear whatever the doctors had to tell us. We left the hospital and our last pre-transplant appointment behind us and headed back to our safe place.

We made it home and called a family meeting. Kris already knew the results of the scan, but Lexi wanted to tell her brother and sisters in person. I watched Cam's face as Lexi told him that the scans showed no evidence of disease. The little girls giggled with delight at her news. I was able to be home and see that in person. We were all together when we told our kids that Lex had cancer, and now we got to be together telling the news that her scans were clear. Although my heart hurt at the knowledge of what was to come, it burst with joy at what had already been overcome. It was a tender mercy I would never forget.

We were due back at the hospital in only a week and a half, and we were determined to not waste a minute of it. Lexi's annual team trip to California was taking place during this time. She was not well enough to go on her own, so we turned it into a family get-away. We drove to California—a ten-hour trip—with six people in our minivan. We've taken road trips before, and like it is with most families, getting there is half the battle. We were prepared for the usual "I don't have enough space" or "She won't stop looking at me," but they never came. Instead our car was filled with, "Hey, have you heard this song?" and "You can lay on my shoulder if you want to go to sleep." I'm not going to lie: it was a little weird. Our kids had always gotten along with one another pretty well, but ten hours in a car can change a person. Even Job would have been impressed with the patience that they were showing toward each other.

I had been praying for months that this trial would have a mini-mum impact on my children. I had prayed that our time apart would be lessened. I had prayed that they would not be changed from the course they were on. How limited had my vision been! I had harbored so much fear for the possible negative impact that cancer *would* have that I had failed to see the positive impact that it *could* have. We had learned that time together was not a chore but a treasure. We had come to understand that most pet peeves don't matter in the long run. We realized the importance of making each moment count.

We had finally made it to California. The Spinnakers were flying in that night, so we had a few hours to kill. We had given our kids the option of going to Disneyland or the beach for that first day, and to our surprise, they just wanted to hang out together by the ocean. We laughed and played, and when it got too cold, we headed to the pier for some dinner.

On our way, we heard someone yell in our direction, "Hey! Hey! She got the cancers?" as he motioned in Lexi's direction.

Kris smiled a bit at his brashness and said, "Yeah, she has cancer."

"Hey, hey, my buddy here, he has the gift. He can cure cancer!" He motioned to his friend, who did not look to be in his right frame of mind. Kris pulled us all a little closer and thanked him for the thought but assured him that her current treatment plan was work-ing just fine. We walked a little faster toward the restaurant and reiterated the importance of keeping the Word of Wisdom to our children.

The rest of the night was spent laughing and joking about things that probably no one else outside our family would find funny. We awoke the next morning and got ready to go to Disneyland with Lexi's team. Our family had been to Disneyland before, but it became evident early on that this trip would prove to be very different from any previous ones. Before leaving the hotel, we needed to make sure that we had Lexi's wheelchair, all of her scheduled medications, and any medications she could need "just in case." Jackets and blankets were packed in case it got too cold, and sunscreen and hats if it got too hot. Heat packs were brought in case of any muscle pain, and ice packs just for good measure.

While we were waiting in line to enter the park, my eyes wandered to a sign that read, "Warning: The Disneyland Resort contains chemicals known to the state of California to cause cancer . . ." Lexi caught sight of the sign and opted to go get a picture next to it, which was then posted on her social media pages with the caption, "Looks like I've been to Disneyland too much!" She laughed ridiculously at her own humor, and we couldn't help but join in.

We entered the park, and Lexi decided to meet up with her friends. She took Cam with her, which was for the best, because he seemed uneasy at the thought of anyone else pushing her wheelchair through the crowded amusement park. So Liv and Aleah got mine and Kris's undivided attention for the next few hours. The day was a much-needed combination of silliness, laughter, and caramel apples. We had planned on watching the parade together that night, and I had been looking forward to it all day. About two hours before the parade was set to begin, Lex and Cam found us. Lex wasn't doing well. She tried to convince us that she would be fine and could just tough it out, but her appearance made our decision clear. It was just a reminder that there is no vacation from cancer.

For the rest of our trip, my mind focused not on how I thought our vacation should be. I focused on how it actually was and how lucky we were to be able to enjoy this time together. We could've been at Disneyland, the beach, or Paris, and it wouldn't have mattered. Cancer would have followed us there. But happiness could also follow us.

The Sunday before we left California was Livi's birthday. She really wanted to spend it eating cake by the ocean, thanks to a popular song. We stopped the day before, bought enough cupcakes for the entire team, and together we sang and celebrated her birthday before driving home.

On the whole, we loved this very special time together, but a piece of me was breaking, knowing how short-lived it was. My mom heart could feel that a storm was coming, and I knew that my children could feel it too. It pained me to know that they had to feel so much emotion at such young ages. The anxiety of knowing that we would soon be apart again sometimes felt like more than I could bear. My heart yearned for the days that they didn't have to ask, "How many more days do we have together?"

We got home from vacation and had one day together before we were due at the hospital for Lexi's first transplant.

Chapter Seventeen

By the Hands of the Apostles Are Wonders Wrought

(Acts 5:12)

*O*nce again we were heading to the hospital, but this time we faced the unknown. We had heard horrors of transplant and what it entailed. I was putting on a calm façade but was trying not to think about the days ahead.

"Ready for our music?" Lex asked. We had established a routine that on each drive to the hospital, we would listen to whatever playlist Lex had compiled to help get her through the upcoming treatment. Some playlists consisted of songs with a lot of fight, some with songs of hope, and some with songs of peace. I wondered what emotions would be revealed in her song choices on this particular day. She was well aware that her young body was likely heading to face the most difficult step she had encountered up to this point.

With that in mind, I was expecting the day's playlist to include hype-up songs to get her ready for battle. The first song came through the speakers, and a peaceful warmth washed over me. "Be Still, My Soul" sounded throughout the car. Rather than sing along like we usually did, we were silent as the music filled our souls.

Be still, my soul: The Lord is on thy side;
With patience bear thy cross of grief or pain.
Leave to thy God to order and provide;

In ev'ry change He faithful will remain.
Be still, my soul: Thy best, thy Heav'nly Friend
Thru thorny ways leads to a joyful end.

It strengthened me to feel the level of understanding that she had been given. In that moment, her faith calmed my fear, and we rode hand in hand to the hospital, knowing that we would not have to face this challenge alone.

The first day at the hospital was spent having a procedure done to have Lexi's port removed and a double lumen Broviac line placed. This was a central line placed in her chest like her port, but it allowed more access for the increased medication that accompanied transplant. Unlike her port, this central line could not be de-accessed at any time. This meant that daily maintenance of the line would be needed until the end of treatment. It also meant that swimming and normal showers would be postponed until further notice because the line could not get wet.

She came out of the procedure with dressing on her new line and steri-strips to help close the incision that was made to remove her port. She woke the next morning to learn that all of her dressings would need to be removed. Just as with the other rounds, Lexi would be getting multiple chemos, one of which, thiotepa, was known to burn the skin through the pores. Any adhesive would greatly aggravate this condition. The next hour was spent with Lexi's jaw clenched as recently applied steri-strips and dressings were removed, leaving her newly acquired incisions exposed.

While doing her best to be gentle, the nurse spoke to us about added precautions that these chemos required. "While this chemo is being administered, Lexi will need to shower three times a day and have her bedding and all clothing washed and changed every time. No one is allowed to touch her skin without gloves for the next several days, because just as it can burn Lexi's skin, it can also burn anyone who comes in contact with her. It's pretty nasty stuff."

The primary thing I had been able to do to offer comfort to Lex was now being threatened. "I'm sorry," I told the nurse, "I refuse to wear gloves to hold my child's hand. This drug is being pumped directly into her heart. The least I can do is offer comfort by holding her hand."

She smiled kindly. "Well, just make sure you wash your hands very thoroughly after and change your clothes often." I smiled and thanked her for understanding.

The chemo hit hard and fast. Lexi had walked herself into the hospital, and within only a few hours after it began, she was unable to stand unassisted. As I held her hand and stared at her quickly weakening body, I could not help but think of what the next several months would hold. I was at a loss. I didn't know how we would watch as our kids held each other and cried at the thought of being separated again, or how we would help Lexi find the physical and emotional strength she would need to get through this. How does anyone "get through this"? I began praying again, for strength, for endurance, for understanding, for anything.

I then came to the knowledge that we didn't need to have the strength or the endurance today to last the coming months. We needed only to muster up the endurance to last through the day. Tomorrow would come, and with it, renewed hope, understanding, and energy. It was easy to look at where we were and compare it to where we wanted to be. There was so much that still needed to happen, but it needed to happen line upon line and precept upon precept. We would gain ground, lose a little, and fight to gain more. Our focus needed to not be solely on the steps that still needed to be taken, but on making sure that we were still heading in the right direction.

Lex was settled, so I decided to head out on my mandated cafeteria outing. I looked up and stopped in my tracks. There was Tracy, Jake's mom. Something wasn't right. We had seen Tracy and Jake a few times in clinic while Jake was getting his labs drawn, and we had kept in touch over the past few months. They shouldn't be here. Jake's treatment was done.

We greeted each other warmly. "What are you guys doing inpatient?" I asked, but the weary look on Tracy's face gave me the answer before her mouth could.

"Jake relapsed," she said simply.

My chest hurt. I could do nothing but shake my head slightly and wish upon everything that I had misheard her. "Tracy, I'm so sorry . . ." was all that came out of my mouth. I'm so sorry? The same response you give when your neighbor has a cold and still has young kids to take care of. I'm so sorry? The same response you give for spilling your drink on someone. That's what came out?

My mind was reeling. I listened as Tracy reiterated the events that led them back here. The only thing that kept going through my mind was, "Jake who rang the bell relapsed. The boy who beat cancer relapsed." This wasn't okay. Cancer should be like the Hunger Games. Once a person beats it, he should get to live the rest of his life like a champion. Enduring this once was more than enough. Why would a person—especially a child—have to fight for his life again? I couldn't comprehend it. How does a mother watch her child go through this again?

My measly appetite was now nonexistent, so I solemnly returned to my room. When Lexi awoke, I held her while I broke the news. Her heart tried to wrap around what she had just learned.

"But he already won. He beat cancer. It shouldn't come back once you beat it," Lexi said. I ached for understanding and how to best comfort her. Right now, she didn't need me to try to fix something I couldn't fix. She just needed someone to listen as she spoke aloud her pain. She asked if I could help her make him a poster to brighten up his room.

"It will probably help him to know that someone understands what he's going through," I said as she was struggling to find the energy to finish the poster.

"But I don't know what he is going through, not exactly," she replied. We began talking about the new friends she had made since diagnosis and how she could relate to them in ways that not many can.

"You have gone through a lot of things already," I said. "By the time you are all the way done, there probably won't be too many things that you haven't experienced. This will help you be able to understand exactly what so many of these kids go through."

"I might experience a lot of the same things, but each situation is different for the person going through it. When someone is telling me about a trial that they are going through, I have learned to not say that I understand how they feel, because honestly I don't. Their trial is theirs and has so many situations that play into it that even if we've gone through the exact same thing, our response to it could be completely different. I just try to listen and offer what support I can. I try to let them know that I love them and will do anything I can to be help them in whatever way they might need me. Really, Mom, Jesus Christ is the only one who can say that He completely understands exactly how we feel."

We finished the poster in silence, and I became lost in my thoughts. How many times had I thought that I understood what someone was going through and thought I knew how they could best handle a situation? How many times had I assumed that because I had experienced something similar, they should have the same response that I had, or would need help in the same way that I did? I did not have to fully understand or experience a situation in order to love and support someone. God has allowed us to develop charity—the pure love of Christ. When charity was my motivation, I could simply express love, take the time to listen, and offer to lighten someone's burden in any way that he or she may need me.

Days passed as I watched Lexi's body become weaker and weaker. The chemo had finally finished, and it was the day of her transplant—her "bone marrow birthday," as they called it. The transplant itself was actually less anticlimactic than the administering of chemo. A technician in a white lab coat comes into your room with what appears to be a very high-tech cooler. The space-age cooler is opened, and a burst of frozen air escapes. If a person is inclined to daydreaming, he or she could easily have come to the conclusion that the same process that is used to keep and then thaw stem cells is also used to store aliens that the government is trying to conceal.

The bag of stem cells are pulled from the cooler and placed in warm water. Once thawed, they are hung and then connected to the patient's central line, and gravity does the rest. The room takes on the strong aroma of creamed corn, and the patient often gets nauseous as the cells enter their body. No pumps are used in the transplant of these cells, because they don't want to risk losing any of them in the process.

Lexi received the transplant, and now all we could do was wait. The effects of the chemo were beginning to manifest themselves, and I stood by powerlessly. Mouth sores had begun to extend down her esophagus, causing chest pain. She had not yet lost the ability to speak, which I counted as a blessing, but it was beginning to take more effort. Her skin began to have a reaction to the chemo known as folliculitis. This means that there was a small infection in each hair follicle on her body, causing small red bumps to cover her skin. Her blood and platelet levels had already taken a hit. Over the past four days, she'd had a transfusion of some kind each day. This was expected to continue for the following few weeks. The doctors were hopeful that by that time her stem cells would engraft, meaning her body had accepted the transplant, it would begin to rescue itself.

In other words, while these effects were horrible, they were also healable. The doctors and nurses were doing everything that they could to keep Lexi comfortable and to minimize her pain. In addition to this, we were surrounded by friends we had made, techs that loved Lexi, and cleaning staff who worked so hard to make sure her environment was completely sanitary. They all became like family. I could feel the genuine love and concern they had for Lexi, each doing all they could do, respectively, to ease her suffering at this time. In the middle of our storm, they brought sunshine to our lives.

Days at the hospital are largely spent doing the same mundane things. The doctors come in and wake you up each morning (usually about three hours after you have finally fallen asleep). They give you the plans for the day and what to expect. They answer any questions, do a quick examination, and then they are on to their next patient. The nurse then comes in and gives you an estimated timeline for the day—how exactly they will balance the meds, transfusions, nutrition, and so on. Then the day is spent either resting, if you are lucky, or trying to find ways to forget that you are in the hospital and why you are there. Wash, rinse, repeat. That's hospital life for you—pretty predictable.

Every once in a while, something happens in the hospital to change things up a bit. A special visitor may come to lift the spirits of the patients. Music therapy or pet therapy can also break up the monotony of hospital living. Unfortunately, these perks cannot be extended to all of the patients. If a patient is on precautions (meaning they have a contagious disease), anyone wishing to see them must fully "gown up" in protective wear and gloves. This inconvenience discourages a lot of visitors. On this particular day, not long after the doctors made their rounds, we got a visit from a woman telling us that she represented public relations for the hospital.

"Lexi, there is a doctor here that is doing research about how elephants don't get cancer. He wants to know why they don't and see if it can help in the fight against cancer. We were wondering if you'd be willing to talk with him about this in front of a camera. We know you aren't feeling well, so please do not feel any pressure." Lexi smiled, excited about the prospect of doing something out of the routine, and nodded.

The cameras, press, and doctor entered the room, and the interview began. It was amazing to hear the advancements that were being made in cancer research. It gave me hope that perhaps future generations and families would not have to endure some of the same heartaches that we had endured. During the interview, the interviewer looked at Lex after hearing everything she had gone through and would go through and asked, "You've experienced so much. What gives you hope in the midst of your trial?"

Her response was simple and immediate: "I'm LDS, so my faith and my family." That struck me hard. Not because I believed that everyone had to be LDS to have faith or appreciate family. What struck me was the conviction with which she expressed it. She knew exactly what she believed, and that knowledge gave her something to hold onto in the most unspeakably difficult times.

I am a person who believes that people need to decide for themselves what is right and live according to their beliefs to the best of their abilities. I believe that family is defined not by blood but by love. I believe that people need to discover who they are and what they believe, and then have the courage to live those beliefs in all they do and say. I believe that when this is done, when we are striving to be the best version of ourselves—whether motivated by a loving Heavenly Father, Buddha, the universe, or anyone or anything else— then our lives and the lives of those around us are strengthened. Lexi knew what she believed and openly lived it. Because of this, she was able to bear testimony and bless lives in the midst of her trial.

Lexi was now seven days post transplant. We had been in the hospital for just over two weeks. Her ANC and white blood cell count was still zero (meaning she still had no immune system), and transfusions continued to be an everyday occurrence. The sores in her mouth raged on with a vengeance. The desire to eat had long since abandoned her, and the ability to do so deserted her as well. The decision was made to put her on TPN (IV nutrition). Her worn-out body had dipped down to ninety-seven pounds, and we couldn't risk her losing more weight.

Her cheeks had begun to resemble that of a chipmunk storing nuts, and it had become extremely difficult for her to speak. She still did it anyway when something was weighing on her mind, but it took much more effort than usual. We worked on reviving our ability to read each other's minds. It proved to not be as successful as we'd hoped, so she began perfecting the art of talking through her teeth. I became fully convinced that if she so desired, she could have a very promising career in ventriloquism one day.

Despite our valiant efforts, thiotepa left its mark on Lexi's skin, burning the lining of her bladder (a condition known as hemorrhagic cystitis), and causing burns on her body where invisible remnants of adhesive had been left. She also sustained burns on the new skin around her scars. The burns were treated by applying cream several times a day. Day by day, they got a little better, and her scars also began to show significant improvement.

I began thinking not only of her scars, but also the scars that each of us bears. Whether they be physical, mental, or emotional, we all have representations of the experiences we have had that manifest themselves in many ways. Before being diagnosed, Lexi had very few scars. The few she had were small and unnoticeable. She now sported several small scars from tubes and drains, ports and lines, biopsies and IVs. These were in addition to the large scar that reached from her back to her belly button and then joined the scar from her rib cage to a few inches below her belly button. To Lexi, these scars were a visual representation that her life was spared, and she wore them with great pride.

Over the past months, Lexi had earned more than fifteen memorable scars as well as countless IV and arterial pokes. Each one of these wounds needed time to heal properly. In order to allow this to happen, she had to follow the instructions given by her surgeon. She had to care for each incision and make sure that she allowed herself to heal. Some incisions required more attention and care than others. Some just needed time, and some needed to be nurtured. As she followed the guidance she was given, the once-painful incisions turned to beautiful new skin, a sign that healing had taken place.

Each of us carries scars. Some are visible, and others we keep hidden from the world. Some are physical and others emotional. However, whatever wounds we may have, we can choose to allow ourselves to heal. We can choose to listen to those who have been there before, those who have overcome similar aches. We can allow ourselves time to care for our physical, mental, and spiritual selves enough to allow healing to occur. As we do so, we will see evidence of a new life—one that could have been lost but instead was saved.

The hours passed like molasses on a cold day, each seeming a little longer than the last. The pain caused by the sores and the weakness from transplant were fully felt by Lexi. Her nail beds began throbbing with pain, and we weren't sure why. We soon found out. As a side effect of transplant, she would lose all of her nails and toenails, and it would take weeks after we were finally home for them to fully grow back.

We knew that in order to see any improvement in her health, we would first need to see indication that Lexi's body had accepted the transplant. This indication would come in the form of her counts becoming existent again and then trending upward. As she was resting one day, I happened to venture out of my room for one of my two daily cafeteria trips. I recognized a voice in the hall that was oddly familiar, and a sense of peace came over me. I knew the voice because I had heard it most of my life . . . in general conference.

My tired head just assumed that someone had the same coping mechanism that we had adopted—that of listening to conference talks to get through difficult times. But as my head tilted to better hear which talk they were listening to, I realized that it wasn't a talk at all, but a conversation. I turned fully around to see Elder Jeffrey R. Holland of the Quorum of the Twelve Apostles standing in the hall. I was awestruck. I asked the nurses at the charge desk if it was inappropriate for me to ask him to visit Lex. I'm not normally the kind to bother someone, especially if they are coming to visit their friends or family, but something urged me on. He and his beautiful wife were now walking my way. If I was going to ask, now would be the time to get some courage.

"Excuse me, Elder Holland?" He turned to me and smiled. I blabbered out something that I would like to think was intelligible, but honestly I was so nervous, I can't guarantee that it was. Lucky for me, he either made sense of my ramblings or took pity on the poor child I was there to take care of, because before I knew it, he and his lovely wife were following me to our room. I entered to find Lexi resting in her bed, her ice packs hanging on either side of her face. This was one way we had found to try to minimize the swelling from the mouth sores. "Lex," I said quickly, "Elder Holland and his wife are at the hospital and they agreed to come see you." Lexi put the ice packs down, and I helped her worn-out body sit up the best it could.

Elder Holland and his wife entered our room and visited like old friends with Lexi as I looked on in amazement. Before he left, he placed the back of his hand on Lexi's swollen cheek. Out of instinct, I jerked slightly knowing how hard we had worked to avoid any contact to her face for the past week due to the severe pain that it caused. I was surprised when she smiled instead of wincing. He then looked at her and told her that there was a special prayer roll for the First Presidency and the Quorum of the Twelve Apostles of The Church of Jesus Christ of Latter-day Saints. "Your name will remain on that prayer roll until you are healed." He and his wife smiled at both of us and left the room.

"Mom." Lexi looked at me through tear-filled eyes. "Did you feel the Spirit when they entered the room? It filled the entire room. Did you feel it? I always want to feel this way." I nodded, not fully trusting that I could speak sensibly yet. She continued, "Did you see when he touched my cheek?" I nodded again and asked if she was okay. "It didn't hurt, Mom . . . It was comforting. It was the first time my cheek hasn't hurt in a long time. It was so comforting that I didn't want him to move his hand because while it was there I knew I wouldn't hurt."

Warmth filled my body from head to toe. I recalled the stories I had grown up learning—the ones where Christ took the time to heal the sick, the time to bless the children one by one. I knew that if Christ himself were to visit our room, He too would touch Lexi's cheek, and His touch alone would bring her comfort. How grateful I was for humble servants of God that lived their lives in such a manner that they were worthy enough to bear record of the Son of God with the touch of their hands. My sentiments echoed that of Lexi's: I always wanted to feel that way. She fell back asleep peacefully and rested better than she had in over a week.

Lexi began showing small improvements each day. Her counts began showing signs of life, and she officially engrafted (meaning her body accepted the transplant). Her mouth sores and the burns on her skin slowly began to heal. The swelling in her face went down, and after what felt like an eternity, she was able to freely laugh and smile again! I could truly say that her smile brightened our whole room. She still needed platelets consistently, but that was to be expected.

Honestly, every time we were told that she needed them, I was reminded of what a miracle it was for them to get as high as they did during her surgery.

She slept upward of eighteen hours a day—every teenager's dream—but the doctors said that it was just the body recovering from what it had been through. She also went through a spell of running fevers, but her body fought to heal itself. We were now on track to go home early the following week. We had plans to be together for about a week or so before coming back for her second transplant, and we felt blessed for this sacred family time.

This wonderful saying expresses all of the things that cancer cannot do:

"Cancer is so limited. It cannot cripple love. It cannot shatter hope. It cannot corrode faith. It cannot eat away peace. It cannot destroy confidence. It cannot kill friendship. It cannot shut out memories. It cannot silence courage. It cannot reduce eternal life. It cannot quench the spirit" (author unknown).

While I loved that saying, I began thinking of all the things cancer can do. It can foster a more genuine empathy and stronger compassion for others. It can teach us to love deeper, live more fully, and laugh more freely. It can show us the beauty that is around us every day that is often overlooked. People appreciate more fully the things in life that have to be worked for. Cancer made us work for every smile, every laugh, and every joy. Because of the effort that was used to find these things, when we found them, we appreciated them all the more.

Chapter Eighteen

I Will Make Weak Things Strong

(Ether 12:27)

We had successfully made it through one transplant and had been sent home to finish recovering and gear up for the second one. When transplants are done successively and so close together, they are known as tandem transplants and have proven to be more effective in the prevention of relapse in high-risk neuroblastoma patients. Being at home was exactly what all of our hearts needed, but just like going to California, it was also a reminder that things were not like they had been before.

We loved being together—that was never a question—but whether or not we liked it, we had to acknowledge the fact that our family dynamic had drastically changed and would continue to remain fluid for the next several months. We had to learn to function together as one but without fully leaning on one another because we didn't know if we would be sleeping under the same roof the following night. It was a tricky process.

We did not master it, not by a long shot. But as we prayed for guidance, we felt it necessary to do all we could to nurture those sacred relationships within our family whenever we had the opportunity. This was not as simple as having a week of family fun, because we still needed consistency for when Lexi and I returned to the hospital. We couldn't leave Kris with chaos, hoping that he would reestablish order in time for us to come home and demolish it again. So we tried to insert Lexi and me into the routine Kris had established without making too many waves. We also tried to pack as much fun in as we could. It was a balancing act, to say the least.

Our home life had changed, and we needed to adjust to it. Watching Lexi suffer physically was a heartache too deep for words, but watching each of my children struggle each day brought a new pain to my soul. One of the most difficult things to watch is the impact that challenges can have on your children, regardless of the challenge, regardless of their age. It became apparent early on that although Lexi was the one diagnosed with cancer, it would affect each of my children in a different way. Cameron became more protective of those around him. He did not like to hear of anyone being picked on or bullied in the slightest. He made it his mission in life to see that no one had to suffer unnecessarily.

Aleah had begun to have the unyielding desire to help and serve others. Without my knowledge, she approached the principal at her school and told her that she was interested in doing a service project. The principal was kind enough to find a project that allowed Aleah to help her schoolmates. She was learning that despite her own trials, she could still look for ways to help others.

Olivia became more compassionate. During our stays at the hospital, we would talk, text, or FaceTime—anything to stay connected while being pulled apart. One conversation will forever replay in my mind.

"How are you doing Livi Butt?"

"I'm good," she responded. "But Mom, last night Aleah was really sad because she misses you and Lexi so much. I miss you guys so much too. I just held her and let her cry herself to sleep. Don't worry, Mom. I took care of her for you. I think she's okay now."

My heart shattered as the image of ten-year-old Livi holding her eight-year-old sister while she cried herself to sleep filled my mind. I didn't want her to have to console her younger sister. I didn't want her to become so familiar with heartbreak. I wanted her to be able to frivolously laugh and play without a care in the world, like most kids her age. I wanted to tell her that she would never have to hold her sister while she cried again. I wanted her to not have to be brave when she was sad. I wanted this to be over, but we had more to experience and more to learn.

I had to refocus. I needed more understanding than I currently had. Right now I was only thinking of my children at their current age. I prayed to be able to see the purpose in their suffering. My thoughts extended to years from now. I thought of not just where my children were currently, but also of the type of people they were becoming. In the midst of this trial, Cam was learning to protect and defend others from unnecessary suffering. Leah was learning that it is important to help and serve others. Liv was learning a deep compassion, the kind that many don't master the entirety of their lives. Cancer would take my family through hell, but it was our choice whether the fire would burn us or refine us.

Every minute and every bit of energy we had became focused on our children and making sure they were as prepared as they could be for the fast-approaching second transplant. Lexi had already been postponed for another week because she had tested positive for E. coli. Her body needed more time and medication to help it recover. The doctors had warned us that they expected her second transplant to be more difficult on her organs and her body in general, so they needed her as healthy as possible before proceeding.

For the past several months, Cam had been working out with the football team at Cyprus High School. Every morning and afternoon, he would lift weights and complete a scheduled workout. One Friday afternoon, I picked him up and asked how the workout had gone. "I'm so sore!" he said. "On Fridays I always feel the weakest that I do all week because my muscles have been worked out every day without a break. But even though I feel the weakest, I'm really at my strongest." I half smiled and urged him on. I cherished the few uninterrupted moments we had together and was interested to see where his logic was going. "I've been working and growing all week. Even though I'm exhausted, I know that when Monday comes, after my body has had time to rest, I will be stronger than I was the week before. I know that if I don't quit, even when I'm sore and tired, then I will keep getting stronger."

His words reached far beyond the weight room. My heart filled with love for our curly-haired son, who was becoming a strong young man in more ways than one. Sure enough, Monday came. He was no longer sore, and he knew he was stronger than he had been before. As we drove home and I asked about weights that day, he said simply, "I was better prepared today than I would have been if I would've quit when it was hard."

I thought of my son and the lesson he had shared with me. If we could just hold on, our "Monday" would come, and we would be better prepared and more capable to handle whatever this life may hold.

The week passed far too quickly, and once again we said our good-byes and then said them again, prolonging the inevitable separation. We made our trek to the hospital for Lexi's second transplant. She received three chemos instead of two for this round. Two of these chemos ran twenty-four hours a day for four days, not giving her body much of a break. The nausea began almost as quickly as the chemos did, so the anti-nausea medications were brought on board. Within hours of the chemo starting, she had lost the ability to stand unassisted, and sitting in a chair was only tolerated for short periods of time. Her body had become so weak so fast. It was already beginning.

Throughout my entire life, I had considered myself an optimist. I still did, but cancer had also taught me to be a realist. Realistically I knew that this transplant would be more difficult than the last; in some ways it already had been. Realistically I knew that with the extremely weakened state that her body was in, it would be more difficult for Lexi to recover. She would do it, but it would be more of a struggle. Realistically, I knew that this would challenge us more than anything had thus far. As I struggled to comprehend these realities, it became difficult at times to not focus on all she was missing, to not focus on how different her life was compared to how we thought it would be.

We had been in the hospital for only two short days when Lexi began experiencing severe pain in her abdomen. I did my best to not panic as flashbacks of the abdominal pain that had led us to where we currently were came to mind. Imaging was done multiple times a day for two days, and a blockage in her intestines was detected. She was consistently getting worse. I couldn't tell if it was the chemo, the pain, or a terrible combination of the two, but one thing was certain: something needed to be done.

A surgeon we had not yet met entered our room. "Hello, Alexis," he said as he surveyed her demeanor. "How are you?" By this point Lexi had found a position that caused her the least amount of pain and was coping by not moving much.

"I'm okay," she responded. "I'm just in pain."

"Well," he said, "you certainly don't look like you need to be rushed into surgery."

Frustrated, I tried to steady my breathing. Rarely did Lexi's countenance accurately convey the pain she was actually in. He did a quick examination and said that he would like to wait until morning to see if this problem would clear up on its own. "This blockage is likely caused by scar tissue from your two previous surgeries that has accumulated and caused your intestines to twist and kink. We need to avoid surgery at all possible costs. The risks that this surgery holds given the weakened state of your body do not outweigh the benefits. I am not willing to be the surgeon to take that risk."

He left our room and my heart sank. I knew as soon as he said the word "surgery" that it was the path we would be taking. We were told that because of excessive scar tissue in Lexi's abdomen, any surgery would be considered major surgery from this point on, and she simply was not healthy enough for that. In addition to this, the chemo she was receiving was hitting her body so hard that within a few days, her immune system would be nonexistent.

A short time later, the surgeon entered our room again. "The imaging from earlier just came back. We can't wait until morning. We need to take Lexi into surgery now. We do not have a choice. They are prepping the OR now." With a small shake of his head, he continued, "The timing could not be worse, but we don't have another option."

I reminded myself to breathe and turned my focus to Lex as he quickly exited the room to prepare for the unexpected surgery. "How are you doing, honey? That's a lot to take in and can be hard to hear when they say some of those things so bluntly." I was realizing that while I appreciated honesty, the mind-set of "ignorance is bliss" was becoming somewhat appealing.

Without fear in her eyes, she looked directly at me and simply said, "I know I will be okay, Mom. I just don't know what I'll have to go through to get there."

I called Kris to update him on the pending surgery. He made sure the kids were all settled and headed up to the hospital to be with us. It took him a mere forty-five minutes to get to the hospital from the time I called him. They had moved so fast in getting Lexi into surgery that he had to meet us in the hall outside of the operating room. He gently kissed her head.

"How are you doing, baby girl?"

A wry smile turned up the corners of her tired mouth as she looked up at her dad. "Well, I thought that fighting neuroblastoma was enough of a challenge, but I guess my body doesn't agree. It thinks we needed something else to tackle." He lovingly smiled at her wit despite the pain and rubbed her bald head before kissing it one last time. The surgeon then approached us along with the nurses, and all too soon we were again left hand in hand to watch our daughter be taken into surgery, with potentially fatal chemo as her companion.

During the day, surgical waiting areas are generally staffed with helpful faces and small snacks to help pass the time. A television is usually set at a volume that doesn't demand attention but allows for needed distraction. But this is not the case during the wee hours of the night. Kris and I quietly walked to the waiting area. The lights were dim and there was no one to greet us. The snack cupboards and mini fridge had been locked for the night—not that food was even a thought at the moment—and the room was silent. When there is nothing to distract you, reality seems to hit a little harder.

A few hours passed before Lexi's surgeon entered the lonely room. "The scar tissue from her previous surgeries caused several hairpin twists and kinks in her intestines—more than I had previously anticipated. I did my best to free them all. The challenge is that by me operating, more scar tissue will likely begin to form. Her body is weak, but overall she is doing well. We will just have to wait to see how she responds. It is horrible timing to need a major operation. You can see her as soon as she is stable." We thanked him, and I thought of not just Lexi's future, but the future of all cancer patients as well.

Generally if a person is sick, the problem is addressed and fixed, and life goes on. If you get appendicitis, the appendix is removed, you recover, and then you resume life. Is this really a possibility for cancer patients? They struggle so hard to survive, yet the cost of that survival comes at such a high price.

The day following her surgery, Lexi's counts dropped to zero, meaning that if any infection were to start in her body, it would be free to run rampant as fast as it could. In addition to the surgical pain, her mouth sores had begun making their appearance as well. During this time, her body needed to be able to focus on surviving until transplant. Instead, it had to simultaneously survive and fight to recover from a major surgery.

To say that it had been a rough few days would have been an understatement. No parent wants to see the look of fear in a surgeon's eyes as he weighs the child's life in his hands. No wife should have to see the look of helplessness in her husband's eyes as he thinks of the child he has vowed to protect, knowing that nothing he could do would save her from the pain that she would have to endure. My fragile heart was brought to a new level of hurt.

I don't know that my mind will ever fully process the magnitude of this experience, but I do know that every time I felt my heart quicken with anxiety or my thoughts grow heavy with sorrow, somehow a peace was able to enter my soul. My grief was overshadowed by the blessings for the future that had been promised, but it was more than that. I had no control, yet I was at peace knowing that whatever happened, we would all be okay. As much as my mind wanted to lash out, my heart needed to hold on, to believe. I could tell that a greater understanding and knowledge had been bestowed upon Lexi as well. In her countenance shone the light of faith, which allowed her to look unfavorable odds in the face time after time and not even quiver.

In the midst of tragedy, it is human nature to focus on one's own feelings. However, this response is counterproductive. When Lexi was diagnosed, both mine and Kris's hearts shattered. There are not words to describe the angst that filled our souls. My role as her mom was primarily that of nurturing, caring, and comforting. I was able to find a small amount of solace in helping Lexi with the things she needed. I could help brush her dwindling locks. I could help her shower and shave her legs. I could paint her nails or help her pick out a new outfit to disguise her port and weight loss. While Kris could have done many of these things, they came secondary to that which he wanted most to do—protect her. He wanted to keep her from any harm, to make sure that she was physically okay. He wanted to fight to keep his family together, to not have to look at the pillow that his wife should be sleeping on and see only mascara stains from where she cried herself to sleep at night. He felt helpless.

It was not that his heartache was greater than mine, or mine greater than his. It was that our heartaches were different. We were a couple, united in purpose but being pulled apart by circumstance. It would have been so easy to focus on the sorrow that was threatening to consume us as individuals, but if we were to divide our emotions now, would they ever fully come back together? Throughout our married life, we had faced numerous challenges, and we had always overcome them—together. This one would be no different. It became a focused effort, despite our own hurting, to check on the other person and ask how they were doing, how we could help. We had to establish relationships and life aside from cancer if we were to maintain them after cancer.

Chapter Nineteen

Health to Thy Navel and Marrow to Thy Bones

(Proverbs 3:8)

*W*e made it back to our room after Lexi woke up and was in good enough condition to be moved. The days following were spent in between restless sleep and exhaustion. The day of transplant had come once again. The doctors and nurses entered our room to sing "Happy BMT Birthday" to Lex once again. This time we decided to make it a little more of a party, because restrictions had been lifted, and her brother and sisters could join in the fun. Jake and Tracy were at the hospital for his clinic appointment, so they came and participated in the celebration.

"We brought you some fireworks and decorations in case you are still here on the Fourth of July, Lex," Tracy said. She really did know how to live hospital life to the fullest. Lexi smiled and thanked her. She then asked Jake how things were going for him.

"Lex," I said, interrupting their conversation on mouth sores. "I'm going to be taking some pictures. Do you want me to touch up your eyebrows?" I asked.

When Lexi first realized she would lose all of her hair, she longingly looked in the mirror and said, "I think I can handle losing all of my hair, Mom, but I'm really going to miss my eyebrows." I vowed to her on that day that she would never go without eyebrows unless she wanted to. She rarely took them completely off, so many people did not realize that they were gone. That was now part of my job description: mom, nurse, eyebrow artist. She nodded and sat still as I penciled her brows in as I had so many times before.

"Wait, what?" Jake said as he watched this exchange. "What are you doing that for?"

"My eyebrows are gone like yours are, Jake. So I fill them in, or my mom helps when I don't feel well."

"Oh that makes sense! I was wondering how you'd kept them so long," Jake replied.

"You know, Jake," I said, "I'd be happy to fill your eyebrows in if you'd like. I'm getting pretty good at it."

He grinned. "Nah, I look good with no brows!" We all laughed at his confidence and agreed with him.

The following days bled into weeks as Lexi's body was again pushed to a place I could only pray it would come back from. Her mouth sores raged on with an unprecedented vengeance.

"My ears hurt so bad," Lexi told the doctors one morning. They examined her ear canals and shook their heads, also noting the swelling around her eyes.

"It looks like the mucusitis has not only extended throughout your entire GI tract but also into your ear canals and your sinuses as well. It's common for mouth sores to go from 'cheek to cheek,' as you are well aware, Lex. But to have them in the ear canals and sinuses like this is something else. They are made of the same tissue that your mouth is made of, so it makes sense, but we've never seen it." I stared at her in disbelief. Leave it to Lex to go the extra mile, even with mouth sores.

Each night we had scripture and prayer. On the nights it was her turn and she couldn't speak, we silently held hands and bowed our heads in unison. When she was finished silently praying, she would gently squeeze my hand, and I would say, "Amen." On Sundays, priesthood holders would come and bless the sacrament specifically for us. This sacred ordinance took on a new meaning as I took a small piece of bread from the tray, broke it (because she was unable to eat the small morsel in its entirety), and carefully placed it between my daughter's swollen lips. She went weeks without eating, but she insisted on partaking of the sacrament each time it was brought to our room. I cherished these sacred moments, fostering a sense of gratitude for our otherwise unbearable situation.

Primary Children's has an LDS branch that meets together once a week for a thirty-minute sacrament meeting. Lexi was not well enough to attend this meeting more than a few times throughout treatment. However, tender moments were still shared. I will never forget the closing prayer to one of the few meetings that we attended. It was offered by a father of one of the patients. He asked God to bless each of the children, and then his voice caught as he humbly said the words, "Nevertheless, not our will but Thine be done."

Our hearts collectively knit together as we were each holding our own heartache, but ultimately we had to turn this over to God. We were being taught lessons. We were learning eternal truths. We were being shown the pure love of God. I have no doubt that given the option, any parent in that room would have done anything in their power to take the suffering from his or her child, but none of us could.

I thought of our Heavenly Father as He beheld the suffering of His Son. He had the power to end it at any time, but more than power, He had the understanding of the necessity of that suffering. He knew that it held a greater purpose that was to be revealed at a later time. He did not allow His Only Begotten to suffer one minute longer than was necessary to fulfill His role in the eternal plan. He would not allow our children to suffer one minute longer than is necessary either. With my limited understanding, I could not fully comprehend why such severe suffering needed to occur at all, especially where children were concerned. However, when I took a step back, I could see the blessings that accompanied such raw anguish.

In my lowest points, I felt more fully the refining Spirit of God. It was not because I held some great power. It was because I recognized so fully that without God I was nothing, I could do nothing. I had to completely give my life to Him in a way I never before had. I was completely vulnerable, completely exposed. My weaknesses had been made bare, and it was through those weaknesses that I gained my greatest understanding of the source of eternal strength. The things of this world are temporary. When we base our happiness on things that don't last, it will always be in jeopardy. Our happiness needs to be rooted in the understanding that joy is an eternal principle.

The Fourth of July arrived, and while we weren't able to make it home, we did get clearance for Lexi to sneak out of her room around ten o'clock that night. I wheeled her around the fourth floor, determined to find the best view of fireworks that the hospital offered. We settled on a small lobby at the end of the fourth floor, and I wheeled her right next to the window.

After I sanitized the window, Lexi put her face right next to the glass to try to get an unobstructed view. As she was watching the silent display of colorful lights, I pulled up Pandora and found an "All-American" music station. The voice on my phone sang tribute to our freedoms, our rights, and those who defend those precious gifts. It was an unconventional holiday, but a beautiful one. Discharge from the hospital came only a few days later, marking a month for this stay.

While many kids were soaking up the summer sun, Lex was preparing for the next step on her road map—radiation. Not two weeks after we were discharged, Lexi was scheduled for her consultation and planning session with the radiologist.

"Basically what will happen," said the radiologist, "is that you will come in every day, Monday through Friday. You will change into a hospital gown and then wait in the waiting room. One of our technicians will come and get you and bring you into the room where you will get your radiation. You will lie flat on your back in the mold we have made of your body, and then we will line up the radiation to the tattoos we will place on your body to make sure that the radiation is going directly into the spot we want it to target. Do you have any questions?"

"Will it hurt me?" Lex asked.

"You may experience some minor burns at the site of radiation. It may feel like a really bad sunburn. You may also feel a bit weaker than normal, and because the radiation is in your abdomen, you may feel a little nauseous."

Lex smiled. "Oh good. If that's it, then this will be like a vacation for my body!"

The technician laughed, though with a tinge of sadness. I loved Lexi's willingness to find the good in everything, but I would be lying if I didn't say that my heart broke a little in knowing that she considered something like radiation to be a vacation when compared to what she had suffered.

As we continued with the appointment, we learned that Lexi would only need twelve rounds of radiation as opposed to the twenty they had previously thought she would get. The more we learned, the more our hearts continued to be eternally grateful for the miracle of her tumor being removed in its entirety. The radiologist reaffirmed that because of the success of her resection surgery, radiation would not be as long and would be more effective in eradicating any neuroblastoma cells that may be left in her body.

The radiologist left, and a technician led us back to the radiation room. Lexi was instructed to lie flat on what appeared to be a highly advanced CT scan machine. The "bed" part of the machine had what appeared to be memory foam surrounding it. Lexi lowered her body down, and two technicians began forming it around her. They worked and molded every curve and length of the outline of her body to ensure perfect positioning for each radiation session. Measurements were taken and charts checked, and checked again.

A marker was used to circle the location where each of her radiation tattoos would need to be placed. After the bed had set, ink was poured onto Lexi's skin in the center of each circle that had been drawn. A small tool that had a needle was placed over the ink, and Lexi was then poked. This process was repeated five times. In addition to her scars, she would now sport five blue freckles throughout her life as evidence of her battle.

The appointment concluded, and we headed back to our car. Lexi spoke up. "You know, I never would have thought that I would get a tattoo when I was fifteen, let alone five of them." I assured her that under different circumstances, she wouldn't have.

The first thing Lexi did when she got home was show her brother and sisters her new ink. Her siblings weren't impressed with the tattoo skills of the radiologist, so we let each of the kids take some markers and turn one of the ink dots into a much cooler tattoo than it was. From that day on, Lex referred to herself as "the painted lady."

Her first session of radiation was scheduled to take place on her sixteenth birthday. Birthdays have always been special in our home, but now they held even more meaning. As this very special day approached, my mind couldn't help but wander back to a year ago and the events and emotions that surrounded her fifteenth birthday. Things that mattered then didn't matter as much now. We all grow and change with each passing year, but it seemed that our family now found ourselves in an alternate lifetime than one short year ago.

There is a saying that many friends had shared with us over the past year. It talked about all of the things that cancer cannot do— cripple love, shatter hope, corrode faith. However, I didn't want to think simply of the things that cancer couldn't do. I wanted to think of the positive things it could do. I decided to consult the wisdom of youth and asked Aleah and Liv to tell me some things that cancer could do. Aleah was first to energetically respond with, "It can definitely take all of your hair!"

This very accurate observation made us laugh out loud, but then Liv responded more pensively. "It can teach us to be a better family and how to love each other better than before."

This journey had taken things from my family that we would never get back. Heartache had been experienced on levels that I previously did not know existed. Likewise, it had given our family things that we would never have otherwise received. Cancer was limited in many aspects but so vast in others. It taught us that life is good but hard, and that's okay, because together we can do hard things. We learned to put the needs of one another before our own and to put aside our own heartache at times to ease the burdens other family members are carrying.

It taught us to love more deeply, laugh more genuinely, and live more completely. I was so focused on cancer not changing me or my relationships that I was missing the opportunity to change for the better: to strengthen relationships, to openly talk about difficult things, and to learn the strength that could come from these relationships. These are lessons that would not have been so deeply rooted without this experience.

Chapter Twenty

He Lends Us Breath

(Mosiah 2:21)

As timing would have it, school began the same week that radiation was scheduled to start. Although she was still in the middle of treatment, Lexi really wanted to start back to school to find some sense of normalcy in her life. Her days needed to consist of more than clinic, hospitals, side effects, and odds. We had cleared it with the administration at her school, as well as her doctors, for her to be able to attend school on a part-time basis. Her schedule was greatly modified to give her the best chance at success.

As I watched her walk into the high school for her first day, a flood of emotions engulfed me. However, two emotions were the most prominent. First, fear: I found myself drowning in "what ifs." What if she didn't have the strength to walk to her classes? What if she couldn't find her classes? What if she got sick in school? What if kids were mean? What if she fell? What if someone sneezed on the desk she would be sitting in? This last one seemed a little extreme, but she had just had her entire immune system reset two months before, and even now it was barely existent. As different scenarios ran rampant through my mind, calmness engulfed me and I was overcome with my second emotion: a spirit of gratitude.

I had the opportunity to watch my child enter her school—an opportunity I didn't know when or if I would get again. I saw her gingerly walk to the door and struggle to open it herself, but she did it. She was healthy enough to walk in the doors by herself. I realized how hard she would have to continue to work for what others took for granted, but oh how grateful I was that she had the ability and strength to work that hard!

Trust me when I say that it would have been so much easier to encourage Lex to stay at home, at least until treatment was complete. She could have stayed in a safe, controlled environment and not faced the challenges she would find herself in at school. I would not have had to experience the fear I had felt. However, in doing so, she would have missed out on so much more than she already had. Sometimes fear is necessary to help us get to where we want to be, where we *need* to be.

For the following three weeks, our daily routine consisted of picking Lexi up from school early and driving to Huntsman Cancer Center. They learned her name quickly and always took us back to the changing room as soon as we got there. Lexi would then change into a hospital gown, and we would wait for the technician to come tell Lexi that it was her turn for radiation. Lexi would then walk with her back to the radiation room while I sat in the waiting room. She would lie in the mold of her body they had created at her first visit, and the radiation would be administered. She would return to me less than fifteen minutes later, and we would head home together.

While having a daily medical appointment could prove to be quite draining, our hearts stayed focused on the fact that we got to go home every day. We got to eat dinner together and kiss each other good night. Our days may have been spent apart, but for this period of time, our nights were spent together—and we even had weekends off! Lexi was right—this was like a vacation from treatment.

With the completion of radiation, Lexi was scheduled to begin antibody therapy in the next few weeks. As a result, she would be getting another full workup of scans and tests to make sure that her body could handle the war that was set to begin. Antibody therapy was a relatively new treatment—meaning that it had just come off a lengthy study proving that the benefits of this treatment outweighed the risks. This step in our road map required that Lex be inpatient for one week out of the month for the coming six months.

During her inpatient stays, she would get an infusion of antibodies that would mimic the natural antibodies in her system, basically giving her an insanely strong immune system. She would also get an infusion of medication that was designed to attach to the cancer cells in her body and essentially mark them with a big target. With her rockin' immune system, her body would seek out those cancer cells with the target and eliminate them—hopefully for good. Instead of causing nausea, like chemo does, antibody therapy was notorious for being painful. They would put Lexi on some IV medication to hopefully offset this effect as much as possible. If scans came back the way we were hoping, this would be the last step—the last six hospital stays—of her treatment!

Time had stood still and yet flown by. Before we knew it, it was September 15—the one-year anniversary of when Alexis was diagnosed with high-risk neuroblastoma. "One year ago today is when we found out Lex had cancer, girls," I told Aleah and Liv as I was helping them get ready for school.

"Yay!" Liv said. "Does that mean we don't have to go to school today?" She was clearly hoping for a party or celebration of some sort. I laughed and reminded her that she had school. They decided on not playing hooky and opted instead to wear their shirts bearing their sister's name to school for super hero day, which just so happened to fall on the same day.

As this day drew nearer, I found a constant stream of feelings continually washing over me. I remembered Kris holding tightly to my hand as the surgeon told us our daughter had cancer. I remembered the feeling of numbness the next day as the doctors forced themselves to sound optimistic while giving us her daunting diagnosis and suffocating road map. I remembered my son doing his best to not show the sheer pain of knowing he would have to helplessly watch his best friend fight for her life, and my sweet little girls doing their best to try to grow up and take on far more responsibility than their years should allow. I remembered hearing the horrors of what treatment would entail and my body going numb because it could not yet process the words I was being told. I remembered combing my daughter's hair like I had a thousand times before and helplessly watching each strand fall. I remembered the looks of sorrow and sadness, of fear and helplessness, all masked behind forced smiles of friends and loved ones striving to show strength for our sake. But that is not all I remembered.

I remembered the beauty of an entire community coming together in support of our family. I remembered Lexi coming home from the hospital for the first time to see her drill sisters lined up on each side of our driveway so that she could walk through Blood Alley. I remembered the tears in Kris's voice as he told me that he came home from a visit to the hospital to find our front yard filled with friends—family—who began singing "Love One Another." I remembered every field Kris coached on and Cam played on that was painted with #AlexisStrong. I remembered all the hugs that were given to my children when I wasn't able to be there. I remembered when Lexi was told through a blessing that we would see firsthand the power of God and the look on the face of the surgeon when he told us that Lexi's tumor had been completely removed. I remembered knowing that God's promises were being kept. I remembered every card, every call, every text, every message, every deed, every visit, and every miracle.

Monday came, as it always does, and Lexi and I headed to the hospital in what was to be the first step of her last treatment. She was admitted to the hospital, and we settled in for the week. In doing a little "mom-to-mom recon," I learned that antibody was especially nasty for the week that it was administered but that once the drug was flushed from the system, any pain or side effects should leave as well. *Five days,* I thought to myself. *We can do five days.*

As promised, when the infusion started, so did the nerve pain. The IV pain medication was already being administered, but the place between enough medication to offset the treatment and breathing on your own is small. Without warning, Lexi began running a fever, her blood pressure dropped to the lowest I had ever seen, and she began retaining fluid. They were able to get her heart rate (one of the indicators of the pain she was in) down to around 150, but then her respiratory rate (how many breaths she was taking a minute) dropped to around a seven (it should be around sixteen). She was on oxygen, but that didn't make her take breaths.

"Sis, I need you to take a breath," I said, not believing how quickly the atmosphere in our room had changed. A few seconds later: "Again, babe. I'm going to need you to keep taking those breaths . . . another one, please." *Five days*, I reminded myself. *She only has to do this for five days, and then she will get a break.* Once we got this medicine out of her body and got home, she should start feeling so much better. She should be able to start regaining strength and going to school—maybe even practice. We just needed to get through these last treatments, just these last few hospital stays.

Once again we found ourselves strapped into the psychological roller coaster, being reminded to keep our arms and legs inside and hold on until the ride comes to a full and complete stop. My head was spinning. The antibody therapy had hit so hard and so fast. I went from laughing at Lexi trying to balance a water bottle on her head and telling me goofy jokes to me reminding her to breathe within a matter of forty-five minutes. It was insane.

Even for those who worked in the medical field, oncology seemed to be a whole new ball game. It amazed me that they knew exactly how far they could push and still allow a patient to recover.

The following days were spent managing side effects of her treatment and praying that time would speed up. The week ended, and we returned to our home, accompanied once more by exhaustion and gratitude. Lexi seemed to still be quite weak but felt that she could walk on her own now that the pain had lessened. A light sprinkling of rain was threatening to dirty our windshield as we pulled into our driveway.

"Are you sure you don't need help getting in?" I asked, noticing that the car had been parked for a minute and Lexi hadn't yet made any effort to even unbuckle her seat belt. "I can come around, or dad can help you inside."

She was staring out her window, and I could only imagine what she must be thinking: missing school, missing dance, missing friends, the pain that the remaining treatments promised to inflict—any of which was worth thinking about. She exhaled, and without saying a word, she grabbed the back collar of her shirt and brought it over her head. I looked at her quizzically, waiting for an explanation or wondering if she had finally just cracked. She shrugged her shoulders and looked at me bluntly as if her actions needed no explanation, but she decided to indulge me anyway. "It looks like it's trying to rain, and I don't want my hair to get ruined by the rain. I worked hard to grow this, and I need to take care of it." I laughed right out loud as she gingerly, but with the utmost seriousness, walked into the house with her shirt protecting her one-quarter inch of newly grown hair.

Our time at home was not quite as ideal as we'd hoped, but we were home, and that was all that mattered. The nightly TPN and the never-ending number of medications (oral chemo was now added to the list, making just over sixty pills that Lexi was taking each day) were all daily reminders that we were still battling, but for now we got to fight hand in hand, not just heart to heart. We focused on the blessing of being together and worked hard to support each other in the small things in life. We found that it really was the small things that mattered.

We headed to the clinic for labs and instructions to prepare Lexi for the next round of antibody therapy.

"Hey, you beautiful ladies!" We turned to see a familiar face.

"Hey, Tracy! Where's Jake?" I replied. We hugged, and I asked what they were doing in clinic as Lexi was checked in and sent to a room. Being a transplant patient meant she would always need to be separated from the general population while at the hospital.

"Treatment isn't going as well as they'd hoped," Tracy said. My heart dropped, and it became hard to breathe. "The cancer has continued to spread. They gave us two options: I can take Jake home and he can just enjoy the rest of his life, or he can start a more aggressive approach. The problem is that they don't know if he can survive the treatment they will need to give him. He still has second degree burns on his hands and feet from the last treatment, and his labs haven't gone back to normal since."

I stood frozen, not wanting to listen to what I had just heard. This couldn't be real. Jake couldn't be going through this. He won. He beat cancer. He was going to beat it again so that he could grow up to be a surgeon, and Lexi could be his nurse, just as they had talked about.

Tracy must have known that there were no words to say, so she changed the subject. "Where'd Lex go? I'm sure Jake will want to say hi." Her question brought me back to the present, and we walked toward where Jake was sitting to see if he wanted to pop in and visit Lex.

True to Jake form, the hat covering his hairless head coordinated with his shorts and shoes. "Hey Jake!" I said, not being able to suppress the smile that always accompanied anyone who was around him.

"Hey!" he said. "Is Lex here?"

"Yeah," I replied. "She's just back in her room. Want to come say hi?"

"Of course!" he said.

"Do you want me to get the wheelchair so you don't need to walk?" Tracy said. Jake was in a wheelchair the last time we saw him inpatient, but many times when a patient goes home, he or she slowly becomes strong enough to walk short distances without assistance.

"No," he said determinedly. "I want to walk to go see Lex."

He struggled to stand from his chair, and I couldn't help but notice the effort it took and the new pink skin on his hands that was trying to grow back. He walked about ten feet assisted, and then we found him a chair to sit in. After he was situated, I opened the door to our room.

"Lex, Jake is here, and he wants to come say hi." She immediately stood and walked out to greet him, and they began chatting.

Jake told us of the care package his favorite singer had sent him. "She put Chap Stick in the package, probably so my lips are soft when we kiss. . . ." He continued, "Yeah, we FaceTime all the time. She can't actually see me, but I can see her."

"So, you just watch her videos on YouTube and call it FaceTiming, Jake?" I asked teasingly, doing my best to keep a straight face.

"Yeah, pretty much," he said, completely unashamed. We laughed at his continued wit despite his physical limitations. We talked for a few more minutes before it was time for them to go.

"Let's get another picture of you two since Lexi has her own eyebrows now," I said. He looked impressed as he touched Lexi's brows.

"Nice, Lex!" he said. I took my phone out, and Lex leaned down and kissed him on the cheek as I took the picture.

"Jake, you are Lexi's first kiss!" I said.

Without hesitation he looked to Lex and replied, "It doesn't count if it's not on the lips, Lex."

"Jacob Bradford!" his mom said as we all started laughing. Goodbyes were said, hugs were given, and we headed back into our room.

Once inside, I told Lexi the news Tracy had shared with me. Her head dropped and tears filled her eyes. "What are they going to do?" she asked with a shaky voice.

"Tracy said that they were going to go home and take the weekend to decide. She wants it to be Jake's decision."

"If he doesn't start treatment, how much longer does he have?" she asked.

I took a moment to breathe before responding. "They think about a month and a half, depending on how fast it spreads. I'm sure he'll probably choose to fight . . . ," I began to say, but my words trailed off when I saw the look on Lexi's face.

"There are things worse than death, Mom."

My stomach grew sick knowing that she was right, and sicker still at how she had come to that knowledge. We waited in silence, both lost in thoughts we wished we weren't having, until the doctors came in to give us instructions for her impending treatment.

In preparation for round two, Lexi would need a constant infusion of medication for the week prior to admission. So in addition to her backpack at school, she would also be carrying around what came to be known as "the fanny pack of inconvenience." It accompanied her everywhere from the classroom to the bathroom. The worst part was that the medication caused her to feel like she had a bad case of the flu. Her worn-out body just couldn't catch a break.

The day for round two to begin was upon us. Lexi walked alongside me as I carried our luggage to our home away from home. We stopped at the double doors to sanitize and then headed in.

"Hey guys!" I turned to see Tracy walking toward us. "I knew you were coming up, so I told them to save you a room by us. You're right there," she said as she pointed to a door, "and we are right here." The two rooms were only a door apart, and we thanked her for thinking of us.

"How's Jake?" Lexi asked, noticing that the blinds on the window to his room were closed—an unusual occurrence for his room.

"Not so good," Tracy responded. "They are thinking of sending us down to the ICU. His body isn't handling the treatments well." She then told Lexi how beautiful she was and asked how her treatments were going.

We settled into our room, and Lexi's treatments began. As promised, it brought with it all of the same effects as before—extreme nerve pain, fevers, blood pressure issues, water retention, heart rate and respiratory rate issues—but it also decided to add a few more effects. Rashes, elevated liver counts, and reduced oxygen levels opted to make an appearance. Due to the high maintenance of antibody therapy patients, each patient has one nurse assigned to just them. These men and women become more than an employee of the hospital. They become family. They don't just care for their patients; they love them. What a unique gift it is to voluntarily invest in another's health, knowing it could end in heartache.

"I know this treatment is important, but Lexi just struggles so much with it," I said to our nurse as I was staring at Lexi asleep in the bed.

She looked at Lex lovingly and said, "This is a new treatment, and a great one, but it is hell. It is extremely intense. Just think of it this way: this treatment is the equivalent of an all-out war taking place inside the body—not just a battle, but a war. That being said, it has been a game-changer. We used to expect that our neuroblastoma patients would relapse. It wasn't an 'if' but a 'when.' Now we don't see as many relapses as before. It has completely changed treatment."

I thanked her for her insight, and she left me alone with my thoughts. I looked at Lexi's small frame. She had been trying so hard to gain weight but currently only weighed ninety-three pounds. Could her body really handle to be at war every three weeks for the next five months?

Despite the anxiety that the thought of the coming months brought, the battle we were going to fight this week was more of an emotional one. Jake and Tracy weighed heavily on both of our minds. This was a side of cancer not everyone saw. A cancer diagnosis causes a person to reside in two worlds. One world is where bad days consist of flat tires and unfair bosses. The other is where children endure the unthinkable in hopes it will be enough, and parents are asked to make decisions no one should ever have to make.

While I appreciated the ignorance of not understanding the cancer world, there was something completely beautiful about it. It was true that this world held a pain and a heartache that many would never know, but it also held a love that few ever experience. It was a deep, unselfish love, one that was motivated solely by concern for others. This world was home to parents who roam the halls sleeplessly at night striving to process the reality of their situation while spending their days doing everything they can to bring a smile to their child's face.

It was a place where people were not separated by social status but united by trial. It was a place where faith and love literally conquered everything, because they were some of the only things that could not be taken. It was a place where triumph came not at beating this disease but by never letting it beat you. A place where small victories were celebrated, a win for one was a win for all, and a friend's loss caused a hurt unlike any other. It was a place where every day was a gift, and miracles were real.

I knew there would come a day when Lexi was cancer free, a day we would no longer have to dry the eyes of our children as they prepared to be apart for hospital stays. There would come a day when we would not have to think about scans, side effects, clinic visits, or central lines. There would be a day where rough days would once again consist of flat tires and unfair bosses. My heart leaped at the thought of such a day; however, I prayed that when it came I would have the ability to always remember the lessons I had learned from the terrible beauty of this cancer world.

Jake was transferred to the ICU later that same day and never came back to the fourth floor. He passed away with Tracy and his beautiful sister, Brittanie, by his side. He will forever be Lexi's first kiss and our hero. We love you forever, Jake who rang the bell.

Chapter Twenty-One

Live in Thanksgiving Daily

(Alma 34:38)

*R*ound two had been completed, and as I was packing up, I couldn't stop thinking of Tracy. She had brought Jake to the hospital and stayed with him so many times, just to pack up and head back home. This time she would be packing up and heading home without her warrior. A sadness deeper than words entered my heart as I silently cried for my friend. We drove home quietly, our heavy hearts comforting one another without speaking. Lexi was currently in between hospital stays, and we were greatly looking forward to the three-week break in between treatments. She was still trying to go to school, but it was becoming increasingly difficult.

"I've heard that they are supposed to recover and feel fine in between treatments," I said to her doctors over the phone. "Lexi is struggling so much in between rounds. Is this normal?" "Normal" is a funny word and one that is largely measured by the situation one finds himself or herself in.

"We only know how our younger patients react to these infusions," they responded. "Lexi is the first teen we have put on this treatment. We really can't tell you how she will react or what the side effects will be for her." I thanked them and hung up, grateful that her symptoms could be managed at home.

Homecoming week happened to fall in the time during this hiatus from the hospital. As the week approached, memories of the previous year's homecoming accompanied it. While Lex was extremely excited to participate in the festivities, she also found herself overwhelmed with the memories of the previous homecoming week and how drastically her life had changed with a single visit to the emergency room. To stay focused on where she currently was in life instead of pining for a life long gone, she set goals for herself. Her first goal was to walk in the homecoming parade with her team and carry her own sabre.

The Spinnakers carrying their sabres in the homecoming parade was as much a part of Magna tradition as the Kennecott Copper Mine. In the past, this would have seemed like a small feat; however, walking wasn't a strong suit of Lexi's these days, and it took everything she had to march every step and execute every sabre command of the 1.1-mile parade route. Upon hearing the words "Ladies, you can break ranks" at the end of the parade route, Lexi turned to me with tears in her blue eyes and said, "I did it, Mama! I really did it!" I ugly cried—again.

Her second goal was to perform with her team at the homecoming game. Since she had last performed with her team seven months ago, she had undergone two transplants, one emergency surgery (in addition to the two she'd already had), twelve rounds of radiation, and begun six months of antibody therapy.

"Honey," I said, needing to ask a question but not sure I could do it without my emotions making an appearance. "I think it is great that you set goals for yourself, but do you think you will really be strong enough to dance?"

Her response came with a fierceness that could not be duplicated. "Cancer did not stop me from performing at homecoming last year. It won't stop me this year."

I knew she wanted more than anything to dance, but I also knew what her body had been through and how weak she still was. On the night before her performance, I grabbed a sharpie and her gore boots. On the inside seam of each shoe I carefully penned the names of fighters we had come to know through this journey. Some of these warriors had beaten cancer, some were still here fighting with us, and some no longer had to fight. The morning of her performance, I handed her the worn-in shoes. She lovingly read each name and softly touched it. She paused and let her fingertips run over Jake's name multiple times as the tears fell freely from her eyes.

"I just thought you could use a little more help today, and these are the toughest kids I know." She thanked me, but she didn't need to. The light that shone in her countenance was thanks enough.

Once again we entered the football field for the homecoming game. Once again we sat on the home side bleachers. Once again we watched our daughter take the field with her team, glittered eyelids and all. However, when she took the field this time, I knew she was dancing for more than just herself. She danced for those who couldn't right then and those who might never dance again. The names of those fighters gave her strength and allowed her war-torn body to perform with the fierceness of a warrior. My heart was full as I watched her dance, not with a physical strength, but with a mental toughness. I saw the struggle it was for her to execute each move and marveled at the will she possessed to do it. She completed the dance and exited the field, her fuzzy head shining under the Friday night lights.

After a beautiful time at home filled with festivities and family, we ventured to the hospital yet again for Lexi's third round of antibody therapy. After this, we would be halfway done with her last treatment. I felt rejuvenated at the thought. We were admitted to the hospital, and again I watched helplessly as my daughter went from laughing and joking with me to enduring more than a person should ever have to.

"All we can do with this treatment is work around the side effects and try to get the patient through the week," the doctor said with pity in his eyes in response to my query of what else could possibly be done to ease her suffering. "This is a little tricky, because we know the common side effects that this treatment will have on a five-year-old, but we are not sure what effects it will have on a teenager. We have never done this particular treatment on someone her age at this hospital." Again the words of the doctor reminded me of the rarity of our situation.

I'd be lying if I said that this knowledge was not a little unsettling to this mama; however, Lex took a different view. She thought it was amazing to have the opportunity to pave the way for kids after her, like so many had done for her. I tried to adopt her outlook and focus on the end goal. At the conclusion of this round, we would have only two more inpatient stays, because the sixth round of antibody could be completed at home. This meant that in as little as four months, we had the possibility of being completely done with treatment.

I was elated at the promise of life after cancer, but I was struggling to find the strength to go on. I was emotionally drained. There was nothing left. I had sat helplessly by my daughter's bedside too many times and prayed that she would come back from where the treatment had taken her.

I had always loved the story of the good Samaritan. It was a story about a man who was beaten and left for dead. Some passed him by, but one man, a Samaritan, stopped, cared for his wounds, and took him to an inn. Upon arrival, the Samaritan paid the innkeeper, asked him to finish nursing the man back to health, and said that he would settle any remaining debt upon his return.

I thought of this story as an example of how I should treat others, thinking I needed to pattern my service to others after that of the Samaritan—observing someone's affliction and then helping in the way that they needed it most. However, my role in this story had drastically changed. I found that over the past year I could relate far more with the man who was beaten and left for dead than that of the Samaritan. I felt as if there had been many times that we, as a family, had lain broken and unable to move forward. However, time and time again we had felt loving arms embrace us and care for us until we had the strength to go on. We had witnessed others' patience as they allowed Kris and me to focus on our children and helped us bear our burdens with loving support.

It was humbling to know that even when we had nothing to give, there were others who were still there to brace us up and nurse us back to health. It was amazing to see the kindness with which we had been cared for. We had been shown love without bias, service without judgment, and understanding without question. Our lives would forever be changed, not just because our daughter had cancer, but because of the gratitude we would forever carry for our modern-day good Samaritans and their countless acts of meal preparation, carpooling, and general concern for our family.

The week ended. Lexi's vitals stabilized once again. We gathered our belongings and took her tattered body home to rest up in time for it to be hit again.

We headed to the clinic to get some routine labs. Lexi was experiencing some intense pain, and that is never taken lightly in the cancer world, so they decided to do some imaging and sent us on our way. The following morning I got a call from her doctors. "We've found some fluid in Lexi's abdomen, and we need you to bring her back up to get more labs."

I got the kids to school, and Lexi and I headed back to the hospital. Labs were again drawn and more imaging done, but this time they needed us to wait until all of the results came back before we could go home.

"Well, we've reviewed the labs," the doctor began, "and there are a lot of little things going on that we do not have an explanation for. Her kidneys are enlarged. Her white blood cell count is trending upward. She has a thickening in the lining of her abdomen. She has lost weight since yesterday, enough that it is a concern. Also, she still has fluid in her abdomen, and we don't know what is causing it."

My tired heart ached, because I knew what was coming next. "With so many little things wrong, we don't know which way she will go, so we don't feel comfortable sending her home. We'd like to admit her for at least a few days so she can be monitored by the bone marrow team as well as the surgical team. We will closely watch what moves her body makes in the next few days and then decide how to proceed." They shuffled out of the room to make preparations for Lexi to be admitted.

This information was more than hard to take. I had taken my kids to school that morning and told them that I would be there to pick them up. They knew we were heading to the hospital, so along with our usual hugs, kisses, and "I love yous," they added, "Come home, and don't stay at the hospital." I now had to tell them that not only would we be staying, but also that I didn't know for how long. I had to hear their tear-filled voices try to sound courageous for my sake, and my heart broke. The last time this happened to us, we were apart for more than three long weeks. I didn't expect us to be here that long this time, but there was no guarantee. My heart pained at the fact that the same heart-wrenching memories of being apart that were flooding my mind were likely assaulting my children as well. Worse yet was that I could not even hold them to offer comfort.

Days before, we had spoken of how thankful we were that Lexi's treatment lined up perfectly so that we would be home together for Thanksgiving and Christmas. No more holidays would be missed because of cancer—or so we thought. That was no longer the case. Thanksgiving was only two days away, and we would not be home. However, if cancer had taught us one thing, it was to hope for the best and plan for the worst. While this was far from the worst, it was a tough day, and no amount of preparation could have protected my heart from this blow.

Lexi was getting noticeably weaker by the hour. No plan had been made, just speculation on what could be causing her symptoms and what would be the best course of action given her fragile state. Currently she was only able to stay awake for about ninety minutes at a time if we were lucky. So we decided that Kris would take the kids to Thanksgiving dinner at his mom's house to maintain some sense of normalcy for them. They would then call when they were on their way to see us at the hospital. I would wake Lex up, have the nurses help prep her and get her ready for transport, and then I'd wheel her down to the cafeteria so we could have Thanksgiving dinner together. We felt truly grateful that she had clearance to go out of her room that day.

Thanksgiving has always been one of my favorite holidays, not just because I love food entirely too much, but also because the focus of the day is on gratitude and family. As I sat in our dark hospital room, there were many emotions that tried to enter my heart, but I was surprised at the emotion that played the most prominent role. Oddly enough, I could not help but be truly grateful. Not just because I was trying to look for ways to mask my sorrow, but also because I had seen so much sadness that I was determined to take every opportunity to look for and enjoy the goodness this life has to offer. I was grateful for doctors who listened to their hearts and nurses who worked on Thanksgiving. I was grateful for hospital staff who recognized that their pillows were horrible, so they brought me three instead of one, and the cashier in the cafeteria who took time to ask about my daughter every time I paid for my meal. I was grateful for the advancements in medicine that allowed Lexi and many like her to live far longer than they otherwise would have. I was grateful for the lady who cleaned our room, who took the time to tell us stories of her children and how proud she was of them.

I was grateful that Lexi's bed was big enough and she was small enough that I could still hold her when she needed me to. I was grateful for a window with blinds that worked so we could see the snow. I was grateful for a daughter who was grateful for everything she had, a son who still hugged me even though he was much taller than I was now, a daughter whose whole face lit up when she smiled, and a daughter who sang songs about how much she loved me and then made up interpretive dances to reinforce that love. I was grateful for a husband who still held my hand like he had for almost eighteen years and could make a Pop-Tart and a trip to InstaCare feel like a date. I was grateful for family who loved me unconditionally and friends who uplifted me. I was grateful for the choice we had to be grateful and the joy that came with it.

I was grateful for a hospital cafeteria that was open and a corner table that was vacant. I was grateful for paper plates and plastic forks.

I was grateful that no matter what else had happened in life, that day I got to spend time with the people that I was most grateful for.

This infusion of gratitude combated the drudgery of hospital life and being apart from my family for the following days. "We should be thankful we have people in our lives worth missing, Mom," Lexi said. "We're lucky to be so close that we want to be together." I smiled at her continued optimism despite her circumstances and did my best to mimic and apply it in my thoughts.

Daily imaging continued to be done to try to find the cause of the mystery pain. But alas, there continued to be little change or progression until one x-ray caught an obstruction in Lexi's intestines. My heart dropped at the news. This was the same thing that had caused her to have emergency surgery during her last transplant. I begged to not have to repeat that horror. Over the course of the following days, the bone marrow team and surgical teams both tried several different methods to try to alleviate the obstruction. A tube going from Lexi's nose down her throat and into her stomach had been placed. Unlike the feeding tubes that she had previously had, this tube was used to suck out the contents of her stomach continually in hopes of giving her intestines a break and allowing them to begin working on their own. Despite the different solutions presented, the problem remained—and worsened.

Night had fallen, and Lexi began experiencing extreme nausea. Throughout the night, her condition greatly worsened. Sleep was abandoned and medications were brought on board to try to help lessen the retching. The pain intensified. The sun rose without any promise that she would get better. Lexi was visibly weaker than the day before and now needed assistance to even sit up. She had become clammy and feverish. Her heart rate escalated, and her pain continued to heighten. Measurements revealed that her already-distended belly had grown four centimeters overnight. Her bone marrow doctors were paged. I could sense the urgency as one nurse called for the other to stay by Lexi's bedside until they arrived.

"The x-rays are showing that the blockage has cleared in one section but has become more compacted in another," they said. "We have never seen anything like this, and frankly, we are not sure how to treat it. This is out of our realm of expertise. We will consult with surgery and bring on the GI [gastrointestinal] specialists to try to formulate a plan." I numbly thanked them as they exited the room. I stared at Lexi's fragile body and knew there would be no way to calm my racing mind until this was settled. I was scared if they did surgery, but terrified if they didn't.

Abdominal surgery was not easy. Anything to do with the intestines was difficult, and in her case, all of the risks were greatly magnified. Due to the nature of Lexi's previous surgeries and the scar tissue that had resulted, any surgery on her abdomen would be a major surgery with major risks and major recovery. Couple that knowledge with the fact that her platelets were still not pulling their weight, and the risks were even higher. And last, the more often she needed to be operated on, the more likely she was to have this same thing happen in the future as the result of more scar tissue. On the other hand, the blockage was such that they were worried about her intestines perforating or tearing. This held serious side effects as well that were, of course, magnified by Lexi's current condition.

I felt physically ill. I could see the finish line. We were so close, yet we found ourselves in another sinkhole just praying to get out. Nurses continued to come in to check on Lexi, give her medicine, and to document her ever-increasing abdomen size. "Really it is just that Lexi wants to experience everything," one of her nurses joked, trying to lighten the heaviness of the emotions in our room. "She is just the ultimate one-upper. There really isn't a lot we do up here that Lexi hasn't gone through. It's almost like she swerves to hit every bump in the road." I tried to muster a small laugh and asked if we could just have a checklist of all of the services that are offered so we could have an idea of what else she needed to go through before we could be done.

Although I appreciated the effort, the superficial banter did little to distract me from the realization that Lexi continued to get worse. She was fleeting, and I knew it. I had been praying through-out the night and into the morning, but I knew that I needed more than my prayers to sustain Lexi through this. I sent out a text and posted on Lexi's group page, pleading that others join with us in praying on Lexi's behalf. I knew I couldn't take care of Lex the way she needed with my mind playing and replaying every possible scenario. I couldn't focus enough to know what questions to ask or choices to make without the combined prayers and faith of others who loved her and would plead to Heavenly Father for her safety.

Our stressful morning turned into a nerve-wracking afternoon. Her belly continued to expand, and she became lethargic. Doctors and nurses continued to come in and out of our room, each looking at Lexi, at her imaging, and back at Lexi. The decision was made that an immediate CT scan needed to be done. By this point Lexi had become completely unresponsive, losing control of all bodily functions. She was transported to imaging in her bed and then transferred to the table for her CT scan and back to her bed, still not able to respond.

Nerves struck my body as I willed myself to remain focused despite the uncontrollable shaking in each of my limbs. I could feel the love and prayers that had been said throughout the day, but I knew she needed more. I got the distinct impression that Lexi needed a priesthood blessing. Kris had been sick all day, and we couldn't risk him giving his sickness to Lex, so we called a few friends to administer to her. They rearranged their schedules to make time to bless our family. Four men who hardly knew each other, but who knew and loved Lex, lovingly placed their hands on her head. Humbly they gave her a blessing.

As the blessing was given, I listened intently, knowing that the purpose of prayer and blessings was not to change the will of God but to allow us to feel understanding and peace in the plan that He has for us. My heart listened as I heard the same promises and blessings reiterated to her once again that had been uttered over a year ago—that she would be healed on God's time and go on to live a very full and happy life. I could not contain my emotions, and my friend who had accompanied her husband put her arms around my shaking shoulders while I quietly sobbed.

How was it that every blessing she had received—each at the hands of different priesthood holders, none of whom had been present at the other blessings—said the same words? It was simply because those blessings were specifically for Alexis from our Heavenly Father. The blessing concluded, and those dear men looked to me. "Emily, would you also like a blessing?"

Heavenly Father had given me answers to everything I had prayed for in Lexi's blessing. Surely He did not need to be bothered with the frailty of my spirit. I tried to suggest that Lexi was the focus and the one that needed healing. I would be okay now, just knowing that she would be okay. They looked at me lovingly and asked again if I wanted a blessing. I was battered and broken. I was unable to recall the last time I had eaten or slept or the next time I would. As of yet, I had been unable to contain the seemingly endless flow of tears that continued to roll down my cheeks, so I just nodded and sat down.

As hands were placed on my head, sacred words were uttered. I felt the shattered pieces of my soul slowly merge with one another and gel in perfect harmony, as if no damage had ever been inflicted. I felt the burden I had been struggling to carry physically lift from my shoulders as the words "He delights in being by your side" were spoken. I was so weak, so feeble, so vulnerable. I had nothing to offer, nothing to give. Yet, the Savior of the world, the King of all Kings, the Holy Redeemer of Man, the very Son of God was delighted to be by my side, lowly as that side may be. Meekness entered my tattered heart as the pure love of Christ healed my soul.

Within an hour, Lexi's belly was measured. It had gone down. Her heart rate and pulse had returned to normal levels. She was no longer feverish. Her pain was present but had lessened. Her eyes began to open, and she began responding to my touch. The doctors and nurses did not understand the change that had taken place. She was not yet out of the dark, but I could now see the light. That night, as it had so many times before, the priesthood of God, combined with the faith, love, and prayers of so many, allowed my daughter's body to do more than she could have done on her own as it simultaneously healed the unspoken fears of a mother's traumatized heart.

A few days passed since that unforgettable night. Lexi's body was still extremely weak, and she willed it to recover once again. As I was helping her worn-out body out of bed and into her wheelchair to get her daily x-ray, she spoke in a voice barely above a whisper. "Mama, I can't move yet. My body can't go. It's too tired and I just can't get it to move. I don't even have the strength to roll over or move my legs. Please, can we wait?"

I knew we needed to go sooner than later in order to check her progress and get a plan for the day. "Just keep your eyes closed and lean on me," I said. "I know where we are going, and I will make sure you get there safely." Trusting me, she nodded ever so slightly, and the process began. I picked her small arms up one at a time and placed them on my shoulders. My arms slid around her back for support, and I helped her sit up. We slowly edged to the side of the bed. Carefully and with much effort, we made the trek to her wheelchair, her body exhausted from the exertion.

At the time, the words I had spoken to Lex meant little. I was thinking only of getting my tired daughter from her bed to her wheelchair only a few feet away, a task that seemed daunting to her. But with my help, she had accomplished it. I was aware of the situation, why things needed to happen, and the timing in which they needed to happen. Lexi did not question and instead just kept her eyes closed, draped her frail arms around me, and rested her head on my shoulder as we walked together. She completely trusted me to get her to where she needed to be.

As the day trudged on, I was reminded of perhaps one of the most humbling lessons thus far. The words I spoke to my daughter continually replayed in my mind, only this time I was the worn-out child. I had always trusted in my Heavenly Father's plan for me, but I worried that I did not have the strength to carry out that plan. Every time I watched my child suffer, every time my babies begged us to come home, every time my husband hurt, I could feel myself get weaker and weaker until even the thought of standing felt overwhelming.

In my mind I felt the need to demonstrate that I had some sort of strength in order to be worthy of Heavenly Father's help. As I was having these thoughts, a picture entered my mind of me helping Lexi. I recalled the emotions that accompanied the event. I was not bothered that she was weak or upset that she didn't have strength. Rather I looked at her with love, grateful that she allowed me to be by her side to help her where she needed to go. I had been by her side this whole time. I had experienced every setback with her. When she hurt, I hurt.

It occurred to me that when I was most weak, when I no longer had the strength I needed to get where I was going, I needed only to trust that I had a loving Heavenly Father who was aware of where I was, where I needed to go, and the timing in which I needed to get there. He continued to be by our side, helping us through our difficult times. When we hurt, He hurt. He understood that I was too tired to understand and saw what my closed eyes could not see. If I would but cast my weak arms upon Him and allow Him to walk by my side, He would safely and lovingly get me to where I needed to be.

The minutes turned to hours and the hours into days. The most recent x-ray showed that Lexi's intestines were still not working the way they should. They believed this to be the underlying problem. The doctors said that this was likely a combination of the treatments and surgeries, coupled with her body being so weak. She just did not have the strength to function. Another medication was added to her daily regimen in hopes of helping her intestines function properly.

A few more days passed and Lexi seemed to be making progress. The doctors entered our room just a few short hours after I had drifted into a restless sleep. They greeted us warmly. They had long since become accustomed to my bed head. "She's on the right path, but we'd really like to keep her here at least a few more days just to monitor her progress." I ventured a glance at Lexi and saw her tired shoulders slouch lower than they had been before. As they left the room, I could sense the discouragement in Lex. We were due back in a week and a half for round three of treatment. We had finally received clearance to proceed, but her heart needed time to recover at home first. It was time to play patient advocate.

"I'll be right back, babe," I said as I stepped out of the room. The doctors were gathered around the nurse's desk just outside our room. "I have a question," I began. "Is there a medically necessary reason that Lexi can't go home?" They looked at me, and I rushed on before I lost my nerve. "She is coming back in just over a week. Over the past few months we have spent more time in the hospital than out of it, and her heart is tired. We live thirty minutes from the hospital, and I will take all of her abdominal measurements and chart her vitals at home. I will even bring her up for daily x-rays. She needs to be home." They looked at me and then at one another.

"I think that actually might be okay," one of the doctors said as he glanced at his colleagues. You do live close enough, and we are just keeping her here to monitor her. You know what signs to look for and when to bring her in, correct?" I assured them that I did and practically skipped back into our room to tell Lexi the much-needed good news. Later that day we packed up and headed home, knowing that daily clinic visits and x-rays would be our new normal for the next ten days. We were okay with this plan as long as we got some time at home. Fighting cancer required a strong body and a strong heart. We did what was best for her heart that day so it could continue to help heal her body.

Chapter Twenty-Two

Lay Thy Hands on Her That
She Might Be Healed

(Mark 5:23)

*W*hile at home, Lexi had the privilege of speaking in an assembly at Cyprus High School in front of her classmates. She had only been home from the hospital for eighteen hours but was determined to keep the commitment she had made. Her body was still in a much-weakened state and was unable to stand for the ten-minute speech she had prepared. A chair was placed in the center of the empty stage, and Lexi gingerly walked out among the applause of the students. I saw her take a breath and knew she was doing her best to calm her nerves and control her pain. Lexi was never one to love direct attention, and now she had hundreds of eyes focused solely on her. She cautiously sat down and began speaking the words she had written.

"Hi! For those of you that don't know me, my name is Alexis Gould. I am a junior here—even though there are freshman that have already spent more time in school than I have. I was asked by the SBOs to share a little bit of a journey that I'm going on with you and the things that I've learned through this experience."

Another purposeful breath as she continued on.

"Last September I went to the ER right after the homecoming game, and they found a tumor in my abdomen that was about the size of a cantaloupe. It had ruptured. They did some tests and found out that the tumor was cancerous. I was diagnosed with high-risk neuroblastoma—which is cancer of the nerves—and given a 30 percent chance to live. The doctors told me that someone my age being diagnosed with this type of cancer is like lightning striking in the same place twice. I am the 1 percent of the 1 percent. The older you are when you are diagnosed, the more aggressive this cancer is. I am the oldest patient that my doctors have ever treated with this cancer by four years, causing that 30 percent chance of survival to drop a lot."

She ventured a glance up, shifted to alleviate the pressure from sitting upright, and continued.

"They put me on the most intense treatment plan at Primary Children's Hospital. This included six rounds of inpatient chemotherapy, where my body would receive multiple chemos each round. There are too many side effects of chemo to list, but memory loss is one—which is why I have to write down everything I wanted to say so that I don't forget it, that and because I get nervous. Hearing loss is another—so if you say hi, and I don't respond, it's not because I am a jerk; please just speak a little louder. Basically, chemo does a lot more than just make your hair fall out—it affects every part of your life. It's just that the hair is what people usually notice.

"I've had three major abdominal surgeries that required multiple surgeons to operate on my body at the same time. My body wasn't healthy enough for any of them. Of these, only one surgery was planned. The other two were emergencies, and I just narrowly escaped from having another surgery recently. After these surgeries, I was placed on life support and spent time in the ICU on breathing machines with multiple tubes and drains going in and out of my body. My insides have literally been on my outsides three times over the past year. It's kind of cool when you think about it. After surgery, my body was too weak to move at all. I needed help to even move my head from side to side. I had to learn to walk again. I had to learn to lift my own arms again."

The room was completely silent.

"Only a few weeks after my first and second surgeries, I was admitted for a stem cell transplant. This treatment includes them giving your body a week of high-dose chemo. The chemo is fatal if the transplant does not take, so they told me that I needed to talk to my parents and let them know how long I wanted them to keep me on life support if the transplant didn't take. The chemo was very intense. Its purpose was to kill all of the marrow in my body, and it did just that. I reached a new physical low and was too sick to even speak for over a week. I was in the hospital for over a month, home for a few weeks, and then the process had to be repeated. Again, my parents had to sign papers that they understood the fatality of the chemo and the risk if the transplant didn't take. Again, I was reminded like many times before, that my life was being challenged and it could go either way.

"After two transplants came the radiation. Radiation was the easiest treatment I've been through. It made me extremely tired and sore. After I finished radiation, I started antibody therapy, and I'm in the middle of that. This therapy specifically targets every nerve cell in my body and attacks any that it thinks is cancerous. It is extremely painful, along with other things. One nurse describes this treatment as an all-out war taking place in your body. I think that is a pretty accurate description."

I listened from the side of the stage, amazed at the composure with which she shared her story.

"Throughout my trial, I have received a lot of support, and I'm so beyond thankful for that. I have also learned some very important lessons. First, I've learned that just because my trial is visual does not mean that it is any more or any less important than someone else's struggle. We all have hard things that we are going through. For me, it is cancer and what comes with it. For others, it is anxiety or depression, problems at school, with friends, or at home, feeling like we aren't good enough or like we've done something stupid and will never quite be the same. We all have hard times; that's just a part of life."

I looked closer to make sure she still had enough strength to finish. I was ready to run out at the first indication she was not okay.

"I've learned that it is not the hard times that define us but how we react to them. When I was diagnosed, I realized that there was a lot I did not have control over. I had cancer. I couldn't control that. If I wanted to live, I would have to go through treatment and deal with the side effects. My choice came in how I would react to the situations I was in. I could choose to be angry and hate my life and the path it had taken, or I could choose to look for the good and be happy. I think we are all faced with these choices. Things happen in our lives that we cannot control. Some come because we made a stupid decision, but some come as a result of the actions of other people. Either way, many times the only thing that we can control is how we will react to a situation. We can choose to be angry and scream that it isn't fair—sometimes it's not—but that won't change anything. We can choose to feel sorry for ourselves and sit around and complain—but that won't change anything either. Or we can choose to embrace our situation and make the most of it. Over the past year I have had many emotions, but they have been mine to experience. The way we feel and react is always our choice.

"When I was diagnosed, many people rallied around me and my family. I was grateful and humbled by the support but didn't really understand it. Kids get diagnosed with cancer all the time. I didn't know what made me different. I am not really a person that likes all of the attention on me, so I didn't really know what to think about it. I realized that kids get cancer all the time, but not everyone notices it. If they were aware of me and my story, maybe they would be more aware of another kid's story and know how to help them. The same goes for someone who is struggling with an unseen illness.

"A lot of times, even when you have a big support group around you, it is easy to feel alone. By sharing our stories of what we are going through, each of us can feel less alone—like someone else knows how we feel. We can change what people are aware of. We have the power to be proactive and constructive in a way that will teach and uplift others. We can make positive changes if we work together in order to overcome our trials instead of argue about one trial being more difficult than another."

Her words were wise beyond her young years.

"I have also learned that regardless of the outside support you have, there comes a time in life when you really have to learn to be okay with who you are. Like a lot of girls, I have always been self-conscious about the way I look. During the past year, this got worse. There was a time when I had no hair and no eyelashes. Cancer has caused me to lose a lot of weight, and I feel too skinny. I really struggled with the way I looked. I had to learn that while I wasn't confident about my appearance, I could still be confident about who I was and what I wanted to do with my life. There are so many times that we are looking for the acceptance and approval of the people around us. It's like we to need to know that someone is always there for us. Even though that is nice to know, ultimately how we live our life and the choices we make have to be up to us.

"I have been lucky enough to have a lot of love and support, but there have been many days spent in a lonely hospital room separated from any contact with my siblings or anyone my age. Maybe the trial you are going through doesn't require a physical separation, but you still feel alone. In these moments, your true self is revealed. When there is no one telling you to smile for a camera, are you still happy? When no one is around to notice, are you still kind? When you are by yourself, are you comfortable with who you are? Like it or not, some of the hardest battles we have to face will be in our own heads. We have the power to decide that we can overcome whatever life gives us. We can choose to be more than our circumstances and to rise above the challenges we all face. We are not alone, but even if we are, we can choose to be okay with that. The power to take charge of our lives and to take responsibility for the lives we choose to lead is inside each of us. Thank you for letting me come speak today."

I rushed out to help her stand as her classmates and friends clapped and cheered for her. I could tell the small encounter had been taxing for her, but she smiled radiantly and shyly waved as she walked off the stage.

Nine days following the assembly, Lexi went back to the hospital for round three of her antibody treatment. Everything went as planned, and we were home by the weekend. The following Monday, we headed back to the clinic for her scheduled labs. The doctors entered our room and pulled up the results of the labs. "Lexi's liver is not functioning as well as it should. Some of her other labs came back a little odd as well," they said. "We feel it is in her best interest to postpone her treatment for another week so we can monitor her labs and make sure she is healthy enough to proceed with treatment."

Her body was exhausted, her energy depleted. She had a yellow glow about her and was as weak as I had seen her in a very, very long time. It was disheartening to accept where we were versus where we thought we would be. I had seen other kids go through antibody. I had talked to their parents. The week of treatment was expected to be horrible, but the few weeks in between, the child was generally able to feel few effects of treatment. This was part of the beauty of antibody.

This just wasn't the case for Lex. I still had an unyielding knowledge that she would one day be okay. I was just not sure what else her body would need to go through to get her there. We left the clinic and began the drive home.

"Mom, it is sometimes hard to think of all the things that I am missing and all the things that I can't do, but I know I am living the life God wants me to live—the life He needs me to live. I thought about it, and do you realize how much we have to be thankful for, Mom?" She then spoke of the Atonement, of faith, of family, and of the undeniable knowledge that she was not alone in this battle. It warmed my heart and refocused my soul. Lexi's body was going through hell, but her spirit was being protected, and I would forever be grateful for that.

Lexi grew ever worse as the time passed. It had been less than forty-eight hours since our last clinic visit, and we found ourselves heading up for more tests. Our doctors took one look at Lex and decided that imaging needed to be done immediately. Her countenance had taken on a yellowish-green pallor. Her feeble frame, no longer even ninety pounds, was only moved with concentrated effort and support. Dark circles had formed under her eyes, which now appeared more of a dull grey. She struggled to engage in conversation, not for lack of desire, but rather for the lack of energy it took to focus.

An ultrasound revealed that Lexi was suffering from gallstones, sludge, and inflammation of the gall bladder. Once again we were admitted without notice. Once again heartbreak stemming from being separated without warning or knowledge of when we would come home demolished the barrier I was trying to build to protect my family from future sadness.

The surgeon that had performed two of Lexi's three surgeries stopped by our room. He had read the ultrasound and was left with no other option. Surgery had to be done immediately to remove Lexi's gall bladder. Generally this was a noninvasive surgery that could be performed laparoscopically. However, like with most medical things, Lexi proved to be the exception.

"Much of the risk of performing this surgery lies in the fact that the gall bladder is connected to a major vessel that supplies blood to the liver," the surgeon said. "If this vessel were to be damaged, it would cause major problems because you can't live without a liver." He looked at us to make sure we understood what he was talking about. He began drawing a rough sketch of the anatomy of the stomach as he continued explaining what Lexi was up against. "It just so happens that this same vessel is one of the many that Lexi's tumor was encasing, making it already weaker and more compromised. Rather than a few minuscule scars, we will need to make a large five-inch incision along her right side."

He tried to apologize to Lexi for adding to her already-impressive collection of scars, but she just shrugged him off. "I like my scars," she said as she smiled softly. "I think they are so cool," she continued slowly and with much effort. "I show them to everyone."

He smiled. "Well to be honest, I've never left a bigger scar on anyone than the ones I've left on you."

She mentally added that to her list of "hospital cred" (that's like medically based "street cred"). "Between my scars, my tattoos, and my short hair, I'm pretty edgy these days, Mom," she hoarsely whispered with her eyes closed. Keeping them open and carrying on a conversation was proving to require too much effort.

I smiled lightly at her humor, as did the surgeon. "Yeah babe," I replied. "You are eighty-nine pounds of pure fury!"

The surgeon left our room, and I called Kris. He made sure that the kids were settled at home and came to be with me and Lexi for the impending surgery. Shortly after Kris arrived, a nurse came to take us down to what was to be no more than a ninety-minute surgery. For the fourth time in ten months we kissed our daughter, held each other's hand, and watched her head into surgery with the risks weighing heavily on our hearts. Hours passed before the surgeon came out.

"Lexi did well overall, but her gall bladder was extremely inflamed and completely surrounded by scar tissue. It was so distorted that it was unrecognizable." He continued with his findings. "The reason the surgery took so long was that I had to do a few things to make sure it was actually the gall bladder that we were removing. It definitely needed to come out. Hopefully now she can start feeling a lot better." We thanked him and anxiously waited for the call saying that Lexi was stable enough for us to go back and be with her as she recovered.

I opened the scriptures on my phone, and something directed me to the "notes" tab, or the place where my highlighted verses were stored. My heart stopped as I read the words: "My little daughter lieth at the point of death: I pray thee, come and lay thy hands on her, that she may be healed; and she shall live" (Mark 5:23).

The scripture was highlighted, but I had no recollection of ever reading this particular scripture, let alone marking it. My tear-filled eyes blinked as I read again the words that seemed to be written solely for my aching heart. I needed the same faith that another heartbroken parent showed so many years ago. There were no words to express my gratitude for the restoration of the priesthood of God on the earth. This sacred power had saved our daughter's life and healed our broken hearts more times than I could count, and it had done it again.

In time, the call came and we headed back to be with Lexi. Although her candor remained, I could sense that she was growing weaker with each procedure. Waking up from anesthetic was not quite the comedy show it once was. Rather, she just expressed gratitude for waking up and the blessings she had, always talking about the gospel and her family and wondering when she could go see them.

We stood by her bedside, each of her hands in one of ours, and I remembered the conversation Lexi and I had on the way to the hospital for this unexpected stay. "Look how pretty the mountains are, Mom. They are just beautiful!" she said.

"They really are," I replied. "One of the most amazing things about them is that from far away the terrain looks smooth, when in reality nothing could be further from the truth. Different colors blend to make a soft scenic picture. The jagged rocks, prickly sagebrush, and dying trees are not visible from afar." I glanced over, making sure she hadn't zoned out. She seemed interested in where my tangent was going, so I continued. "However, neither are the wildflowers that spontaneously grow. Sometimes in life we have to walk through rough terrain to enjoy the beauty of the wildflowers." I smiled a melancholy smile.

"What are you thinking about, Mama?" Her voice brought me back to the present, and I smiled as I squeezed her hand.

"Just thinking about all of the wildflowers we've found along our path through this journey," I said wistfully. "My favorite thing about wildflowers is that to me they are pure evidence of God. No one plants the flowers in the mountains. No one makes sure they have enough light or enough water to properly grow. It is all natural. God allows them to grow so I can appreciate them. He knows I love flowers, and it reminds me that I matter to Him."

"I really love wildflowers. I can't wait until we can go camping together again and see some," she said sleepily.

"Me too, baby girl. Me too."

Chapter Twenty-Three

My Heart Was Lifted Up with Gladness

(D&C 19:39)

*K*ris helped us get settled back in our room on the fourth floor and then headed home in time to pick the kids up from school. Lexi was beyond exhausted and in an extreme amount of pain, but her heart continued to remain strong, and we were thankful for that. It was nearing Christmas once again, and we had yet to receive word of when we would be able to go home. Lexi's fourth round of antibody therapy was scheduled to begin on December 26, and we were just praying that we would get at least a few days together before then.

Abdominal surgery was difficult because they quite literally cut through the muscles needed to power movement in your body. Lexi knew that if she wanted to go home, she would have to show them she could walk. She didn't waste any time. She went on her first walk not twenty-four hours after surgery. This was done by me helping her sit in her bed, her working extremely hard to scoot her eighty-nine-pound body the few inches to the side of her bed, and then after taking the time to recover from the exertion, me helping her stand. From there, she and I grasped one another's elbows, and she leaned against my body for support. It was a very painful process, and the farther she went, the worse the pain grew.

Her feet slowly shuffled across the floor, each step moving us only three inches closer to our goal. I could feel her body tense up from the pain, and she began to shake. Her shoulders drooped, and her grip on my elbows tightened. She was hurting bad. Her head still leaned on my shoulder. The strength to hold it up on her own wouldn't return for a few days. I could feel her jaw clench and tighten as she continued to push forward. I held tighter to her elbows and did all I could to support her frail body against mine.

Just as I thought she would ask if we could go back to our room, she spoke. In a hoarse whisper, she said, "Your shirt is helping me so much." I looked down and realized I was wearing my Jake shirt that we had made for his celebration of life not long ago. She had been focusing on his name to help her take each step. She could feel him with her, cheering her on and reminding her that she could do this. Tears fell down my cheek, and I knew he continued to fight alongside her.

The following day, she walked five feet farther than she had the previous day. Restrictions had changed, allowing all of the kids to come visit, and we couldn't have been more grateful. Kris and the kids came up, and Lexi was able to sit up long enough to go to the cafeteria to play games for almost an hour. It was a welcome break from the scenery of our hospital room and the conversations that were taking place there.

Because of Lexi's continuing weight loss, it was decided that she would again need a feeding tube. In spite of her attempts to eat as much and as often as she could, her body was still losing weight. She had become gaunt, and despite the fact that she was supposed to be heading in a positive direction, it was clear to see she was not.

"The issue we are having," the doctors said, "is that her body is no longer processing nutrients and calories the way it needs to. There is no way she will be able to come back from this on her own. She will be getting nutrition twenty-four hours a day and still needs to eat as much as she can. We know this isn't what she wanted, but we feel that overall it will give her a big boost on her road to recovery. We just really need to see improvement at this stage, and we have yet to see it." Lexi nodded that she understood and did the best she could to adapt to her new accessory.

Christmas was less than two weeks away, and there was still no indication of whether we would be together. Like many families, every year we have each of our kids make a Christmas list of the things they would like the most. At the top of Lexi's list in all caps were the words "BE HOME!!" It was not the typical Christmas wish for a sixteen-year-old girl, but she had seen enough in her young life to know what was truly important.

The days continued to pass us by with little notice. We were told that Lexi would likely be ready to go home by the beginning of the week, only to be told that we should be fortunate to get out by the weekend. My heart was exhausted. I could see Lexi getting a little better each day. She was still very weak, and pain was a constant companion, but overall she was doing better than before. I felt we had taken her home in worse condition than she was currently in, so I couldn't understand why they kept pushing us back. Each day our kids asked Kris and me when Lexi and I could come home and we could all be together. Each day we were unable to give them a positive answer. Each day we heard the crack in their voices as they tried to be brave in uncertainty. It was more than a heart could take.

I was getting ready to demand a medically necessary reason for our stay when my daughter once again taught me a valuable lesson. Lexi and I were on our daily walk. Slowly she had become strong enough to need my arms only for balance as opposed to support. Occasionally, to impress the nurses or her dad, she would let go of my arms for a brief moment as if to say, "Look! No hands!" only to quickly grab them again to steady herself. As we were walking, my mind was formulating the conversation I would have with the medical team in hopes of breaking us out of there sooner than later.

"Mom," she said, "I'm not sure why, but I just thought of the words from the blessing Dad gave me right before this surgery. Do you remember what it said? It said, 'Listen to your doctors.' I really don't want to listen right now when they say that I need to stay longer. I'm really tired of the hospital and I want to go home, but maybe they know something that we don't know. Maybe something is going to happen that I'll need to be here for."

My heart was filled with humility, a common occurrence these days. When Lexi came in to the hospital over two weeks ago, she was extremely ill, and for probably the first time since diagnosis, her countenance matched how she was feeling. She weighed eighty-nine pounds dressed in a hoodie and sweats. Her skin and the whites of her eyes were jaundice. Dark circles had taken residence under her sunken eyes, and walking was only accomplished with much effort. The medical team said that she had looked worse than they had ever seen her. As Lexi reminded me of the blessing she had been given, I was able to focus on the fact that these doctors had and continued to have what was best for Lexi in the forefront of their minds.

Once again my heart softened. While my yearning for us to be together didn't lessen, my heart refocused on trusting what I had already been taught. We knew that we had been blessed by following the guidance we had received through the power of the priesthood. We had been shown that prayers were always answered—not always on our time frame or how we wanted, but always how we needed. I was so grateful for this reminder and the peace that came as my frustration turned to trust.

Three days later, the doctors came in and said that Lexi had made some great progress. They felt comfortable sending her home. They would move her next round of antibody back a week, allowing us a small break. Lexi would get her Christmas wish, and the prayers of my children were answered. We would spend the next ten days under the same roof. The greatest part was that she would be released on the day of her sisters' Christmas sing-along. Another Christmas surprise was already in place.

The nurse raced to discharge us, and we quickly loaded the car. I had told the girls that I would do my best to make it to the Christmas sing-along, but if I couldn't, then their dad would be there. Given our situation, we couldn't make promises that we might not be able to keep. Never in their dreams would they have expected that Lexi would be there.

We quickly parked the car, and I unloaded the wheelchair, knowing that Lexi was far too weak to walk. We entered the elementary school gymnasium just as the first grade was finishing their carol. Some friends who knew we were coming had saved us a few seats on the front row. I parked Lexi next to a chair and sat down. Cam had been picked up by his uncle and met us there. We watched with anticipation as each grade entered, sang the songs they had practiced, and exited the stage.

Fourth grade was up next. We watched excitedly as the kids piled in, trying to not trip over each other while locating their parents. I saw Aleah enter the gym and scan the area, looking for us. I raised my hand and formed the "I love you" symbol in the air. Her eyes caught our sign and she beamed. She then realized that Cameron was sitting next to me, and then her eyes moved to the wheelchair next to him. Her face broke into a smile that was so wide, I wondered if it would stay like that permanently. She sang her heart out, and when it was over, she just smiled and stared. I motioned for her, letting her know that it was okay to come and hug us before she went back to class. Without hesitation she ran to us and jumped in my arms. Knowing that Lexi wasn't quite as durable, she carefully leaned over and hugged her. Her young blue eyes watered, and she hugged each of us again before heading back to class.

The fifth grade entered and sang their songs, giving me an opportunity to compose myself. They finished and exited the gym and the sixth graders began filing in. Butterflies filled my stomach as I watched for Livi's tall frame. This was her last elementary sing-along, and she was planning on giving Lexi a full show at the hospital later that day. She entered, and like Aleah, she looked around until she saw me. Her eyes immediately fell on Lexi, and her entire face lit up. She was so excited that she couldn't stand still. The music started playing, and she stared straight at her sister and sang the words she had practiced.

She got through the first two lines of the Christmas song and the emotion took over. Her smile broke, her lip began to quiver, and tears spilled from her green eyes. I stood and rushed to her side. She crashed into my body and started sobbing. I took her freckle-filled face in my hands, and she smiled with tear-stained cheeks. "Mom, I've just missed you guys so much! I just can't believe that you are really here! You guys are home! You get to be home for Christmas? Lexi too?! You're really here!"

I wiped her bright eyes. "We are here, honey, and we get to be here for Christmas. All of us will be home together. You get to sing to Lexi right now, not in a hospital room. Do you want to finish singing the songs you worked so hard on?" She nodded and took my hand in hers. She turned back around. She did not face her teacher or the audience. She was singing directly to her sister.

She continued to grasp my hand and sang every word of her songs. I knelt behind her and silently sobbed, thanking God once again for our Christmas miracle. Upon completion of the carols, Livi broke ranks and ran to her sister's wheelchair. "I've just missed you so, so much Lex!" she said as more tears were spilled by all who witnessed the embrace. Livi turned to go and looked back at her sister. "Oh, Lex?"

"Yeah?" Lexi said, smiling.

"You look beautiful today."

Lexi's tired smile broadened. Since the day that Lexi had lost her hair, Livi had made it her personal mission to tell Lexi every day that she looked beautiful. The message had been delivered via FaceTime, text, or handwritten card. Today it got to be delivered personally.

Chapter Twenty-Four

We Are Not the Only Ones to Suffer

(1 Peter 3:18)

*C*hristmas was spent in the comfort of our home, enjoying the miracle that we had the opportunity to be together. Breakfast in bed happened once again, and this time Cam and Lex invited Liv to be a part of the tradition. She was ecstatic at being considered one of the big kids. Presents were opened, and family time enjoyed. I couldn't help but recognize how frail Lexi looked. Over the past month or so, her body had begun to more fully feel the harsh effects of her treatment. She walked with more effort and struggled to stand. She often needed to rest, even after riding in a car. Oftentimes people had only seen Lexi when she had been well enough to go out of the house, or when she was lying on the couch. During this time she continued to smile and carry on conversation when she could, but there was no denying that she had been getting consistently weaker. She allowed few to know exactly how sick she had become.

Over the course of the previous months, we had not had ten consecutive days at home. We had a goal to break that record, but that would not happen this time. Nausea took over, and as I watched her lying on the couch vomiting one feeding tube after another, I knew this was one record that wouldn't be broken this week. Two days after Christmas, we headed back to the hospital. I had placed feeding tube after feeding tube, and her body continued to reject them. She was getting worse. We were admitted at the sight of Lexi, since her doctors noted that her body was in the worst condition they had ever seen it in.

She had lost four pounds in just six days. Fully clothed, she weighed in at eight-five pounds. Her body was rejecting the nutrition she was receiving through the feeding tube, and she had been unable to eat. They did an X-ray and a CT scan and found that she had SMA syndrome. In layman's terms: the beginning of her small intestine was squished between two arteries. Her feeding tube wouldn't work because the nutrition would enter the stomach but could not be processed and passed through the intestines.

She also had focal inflammation in her small intestine and large intestine. "We know that she is scheduled to begin treatment again on Monday," the doctor said, "but that can't happen. She will not be able to survive the intensity of it until this problem is resolved. We feel it is necessary to scope her entire digestive tract. We will be looking for any additional problems or any evidence of disease that perhaps was lying dormant all this time."

I couldn't believe this was happening. We were supposed to be on the downhill side of treatment. Our hard days were supposed to be behind us, yet we found ourselves facing another uphill climb.

The doctor continued. "We are not expecting to find any new disease, but we want to be certain. Everything about Lexi has been an enigma, and we need to be sure we are not missing anything." That did little to calm my pulsing nerves. While the doctors were asking if I had any questions or concerns (I did, but nothing I dared voice for fear of breaking down), a gastrointestinal specialist entered our room.

"I have reviewed Lexi's imaging and her files. You've had quite the rough road, young woman," he said as he looked from me to Lexi. She weakly tried to smile but couldn't muster the energy it took. "I'd like to place a GJ tube." He grabbed a dry erase marker and drew the digestive tract on the mirror in our hospital room. I vaguely remembered a time when mirrors were used for something other than drawing my daughter's anatomy on. He continued with his explanation.

"This is a combination of two feeding tubes. The first, a J tube, will bypass her stomach and the problem area and put nutrition directly into her intestine. Once her body can handle that, she will graduate to using the G tube, which will put nutrition directly into her stomach, and then her stomach will pass it through to her intestines and on down the line. These tubes are placed surgically and can usually be done laproscopically. That's not the case for Lexi. Her past medical history brings higher risk and longer recovery time with it. However, if we can place it, this should counteract the SMA and help her begin to gain weight and heal."

I felt a sick sense of déjà vu. I swear I had just had a medical professional tell me that my daughter needed surgery and that it typically was a small procedure but in her case would be a major one. Why couldn't I have déjà vu about being in Disneyland? I thanked him for his time and turned back to look at Lexi's fragile body. She had found a comfortable position and was resting again. The brief interaction with the medical team had burned what little energy she had. As I gazed at her, I allowed my thoughts to wander.

Before we came in on Tuesday afternoon, Lex was sitting on the couch watching me put away Christmas decorations. She had been getting progressively sicker throughout the day, and I had been on and off the phone with the doctors formulating a plan. Out of the blue, she weakly said, "Mom, do you ever have those times where you just look around at your life and you are just so thankful? I mean, I'm grateful for my life everyday, but sometimes it just hits me how blessed I am that it feels like my heart can't hold it."

I felt like I had just been hit by a train. It had been more than a month since Lexi had been able to walk unassisted. I had spent the last few nights holding her while she tried to alternate between retching and sleeping, yet she was telling me how grateful she felt. If I were to be honest, gratitude was not the prominent emotion I had been experiencing. My heart was heavy as I pondered on how much longer we would have to watch our child suffer, what else would she lose, and how much more she could endure. With treatment being almost complete, she should be getting progressively better, but the opposite was true.

I remembered our most recent trip to the hospital. Lexi was too worn out to play DJ. Instead, she remained focused on having her blue vomit bag close. I spent the quiet drive alternating between praying for understanding and asking why now, when she was physically at her very weakest, was my daughter being tried so relentlessly? Hadn't she already gone through enough? At this moment, two thoughts entered my mind. First, I thought of the life of Christ and realized that He was tried and tested after He had fasted for forty days—when He was physically at His weakest. Immediately following came the words "The Son of Man hath descended below them all. Art thou greater than He?" (D&C 122:8).

My head hung and my murmuring ceased. How many times had I asked to be more like Christ? How many times had I professed to give anything to become more like Him? My trials were nothing compared to what He endured, yet my feeble heart groaned under the weight. I realized that this was not a contest. It was not that I had to endure everything Christ did in order to become like Him. It was merely that I was being asked to endure the few trials I had in the same manner that He had. He had overcome the world. I didn't have to. We could overcome because He first overcame, and He did so willingly.

Our week had been filled with testing and imaging. Lexi's brittle body was moved from one machine to her bed or wheelchair, only to be moved to another machine. Imaging often had to be stopped or cut short due to the excessive vomiting. Overall it had been uneventful, which, when it came to the cancer life, was both good news and difficult news. The good news being that nothing had gotten worse. The difficult news was that nothing had gotten better. Every day we would see at least one representative from the bone marrow, surgical, and GI teams in addition to any other specialists they felt would be a benefit in solving Lexi's case.

"Lexi is an enigma," the doctor stated plainly. "We know what is wrong, but no one knows how to fix it. We are really good at breaking things around here, not so good at fixing them. Her body is shutting down. Her body is not accepting or processing nutrients. This is likely a combination of the results of treatment and the surgeries. She has so many extenuating circumstances that have to be taken into consideration. Right now Lexi is stuck in a horrible cycle, and we are looking for the safest possible way to break that cycle." Essentially, we were using Band-Aids to fix bullet holes.

Many helpful souls reached out and asked why we didn't just have Lexi eat a cheeseburger and a shake. "Surely that will help her gain the weight back!" they would say, half jesting. While I truly wished it were that simple, it was not. Lexi could eat and swallow food, but when it tried to enter her small intestine, it wouldn't go through. Instead, it would cause extreme nausea, pain, general complications, and ultimately result in retching. We were stuck in the definition of insanity—Lexi was determined to continue to repeat the same process over and over, praying that she could will her body to accept the nutrition, but ultimately the outcome was the same time after time. We would be residing in the hospital until a concrete plan and adequate progress in the right direction could be made. No answers, no time frame, no end in sight.

It was clear that cancer robs a person of parts of their life that they will never get back and then steals things from them that others cannot see for years to come.

When you think about it, we all have some form of cancer in our lives. We all have something that we are striving to get rid of to make our lives a little better. Depression, anxiety, hatred, addiction, and so on, are all forms of a cancer that is threatening to consume us if we do nothing to counteract it. These cancers may not be as evident on physical scans but can be just as damaging. Just as Lexi needed to be treated by professionals who knew and understood her case, we, too, need the help and guidance of someone who knows and understands our individual needs and situations. Ultimately it comes down to doing whatever needs to be done in order to become the healthiest version of ourselves for the ones we love.

Days dragged on, and my mind shifted into overdrive, trying to learn and process something—anything. It wouldn't shut off—it couldn't. My trips to the cafeteria were spent walking the same route trying to expel the stress from our situation through the soles of my worn-out Nikes. I tried to switch gears. I couldn't think of how I would solve Lexi's situation. It would be like trying to win a game of solitaire with only forty-nine cards. I knew she would get through this, just not when. I couldn't struggle through this quicksand. It was too emotionally exhausting. I just had to wait until someone came along with a vine to pull us out.

During the difficult times, I strived to stay focused on the blessings we had received and the miracles we had seen. I found that it helped me remain grateful despite our current surroundings. We had once again found ourselves in a challenging position. I often thought of the miracles Christ performed when He was on the earth. I had thought about how amazing it would have been to be the mother of a child who sat on His lap and was blessed by His hands, the wife of the blind man he healed, or the sister of the boy he raised from the dead. This time, instead of the miracles themselves, I thought of the lives of these people before and after the miracles. The children did not have carefree lives before being held in the arms of the Savior, the man spent his entire life blind, and the sister watched her brother die, all before the miracles happened.

Furthermore, we do not know much about the long-term lives of the people who witnessed these miracles first hand, but I believe they did not go on to never feel heartache again. Challenges would continue to come. That was part of life. Just because we have an umbrella does not mean it will never rain—only that we will be somewhat protected from the full effects of the storm.

Night was once again upon us, and Lexi had fallen asleep. Many of her days and nights were spent sleeping lately, simply because being awake required too much energy that her body did not have. The quietness of the night did nothing but allow my mind to more fully scream the reality that we were facing. My eyes closed just to replay the events of the previous days. Images of the effort it took for Lexi to move her emaciated frame, with my assistance, the short distance from her bed to the shower in her room, and the price of recovery she would inevitably pay afterward, each took a turn in their relentless assault of my psyche. The skeletal appearance of her hands in mine, the withered look in her eyes—the transformation was undeniable, yet I refused to accept it.

Rather than lay sleepless in my bed, I opted yet again to walk the halls of the hospital, trying to process our situation. On my way out of the room, our nurse stopped me. "Have they come up with a plan yet?" she asked, knowing the seriousness we were facing.

"Not yet. They just don't know what to do." She looked at me with empathy in her eyes, and I went on. "I'm sure I am just over-reacting, but I am worried. I am really worried." I cleared my throat and steadied myself. "I have seen kids look better than Lexi looks right now, and they didn't even make it a month. I'm sure it is just lack of sleep and over-thinking, but I can't get my mind off of it."

My fears continued to roll from my tongue like a poison that I couldn't spit out fast enough. "She is getting weaker—lethargic. She doesn't have much energy or a desire to do anything. She can no longer sit up, and when I help her shower, I can count each of her ribs clearly, front and back. Her hips protrude greatly, and I can see both bones in her shoulders. Honestly, I feel like I can see each bone in her body. She has no fat left. Every day they weigh her, and every day my heart breaks a little more. She continues to lose weight, and her 5'7" frame now weighs only eight-four pounds. They don't even want me taking her on walks right now because it could burn calories, and she doesn't have anything to burn. If she continues like this, the malnutrition will start taking its toll on her heart and vital organs. She tries so hard to eat. She just won't quit. She eats and her body rejects it, every time. I just don't know what to do."

She listened to every word I said before choosing her response purposefully. "Emily, I am very concerned too. You are not over-reacting. The stage Lexi's body is in should not be taken lightly. Her body has quit. It has had enough and has literally shut down. Lexi's heart is the only thing fighting right now, because there is no physical way her body could be. Her heart, her will to fight, is the only thing keeping her alive. A solution needs to be found sooner than later—before her heart has had enough. If her heart quits, there is nothing else that will be able to be done."

I dazedly thanked her for validating my concerns, but I was not fully sure that I wanted them validated. It would have been nice to be told I was overreacting, even though I knew in my heart that I wasn't.

Needless to say, that night was not a good one for sleep. I paced through the hospital halls only to come back to our room and hold Lexi's frail frame in my arms. As I cradled her scrawny shoulders, I silently urged her heart to keep fighting. I pleaded throughout the night for guidance on how to proceed. We were at a crossroads, and I was not equipped to know which path to take. Kris and I had decided that action needed to be taken, something needed to happen. We did not know exactly what to do, but we could no longer stand idly by while she was actively getting worse. The morning dawned, and I requested a care conference with the teams of doctors that were trying to help Lexi. I met with a lot of people a lot smarter than I was and tried to collect my thoughts.

"We need a plan," I began, willing myself to remain calm enough to voice my concerns in a logical manner. "Lexi has been getting consistently worse for the past two weeks, and something needs to be done. I don't know what exactly, but my daughter's body has been broken, and I need to know how we are going to fix it."

They looked at one another, slightly taken aback, and began offering ideas. A G-tube (a small feeding tube inserted directly into the stomach) was the first choice from the GI specialist but was quickly dismissed by the surgeon, stating that Lexi's last surgery revealed that the buildup of scar tissue in her abdomen was so severe that her stomach was not even recognizable. Thus, while a G-tube would be a minor surgery for most, it would be a major surgery with major recovery and complications for Lexi, to the point that our surgeon would not sign off on the surgery or allow his staff to do so.

Okay, then. Moving on.

Next, it was suggested that we could give Lexi IV nutrition (TPN) like she'd had in the past. The problem with this is that she did not have the central line space to receive the amount of TPN she would need and finish out her remaining antibody therapy. Additionally, TPN is not natural, and the body knows it. It is not a long-term solution but a temporary fix. Lexi's body had already been on it for extended periods of time throughout treatment. Her liver and kidneys were already showing signs of the wear and tear from treatment and previous use. Now we were going to expose them further to TPN. This didn't seem like the best plan.

Next.

Finally a plan was made that hinged on an NJ tube (a tube that leads from her nose directly to her jejunum—a place in her small intestine) being placed under sedation. It was decided that this would happen later that day, and by that night we should see hopeful progress. Fingers crossed for no weight loss the following morning for the first time in weeks. They called in the best of the best interventional radiologists to perform the small procedure. But, after two hours and two doctors, their efforts proved to be in vain. Lexi's anatomy was such that they would not be able to place the tube. We were at a loss. This was plan A, B, and C.

We took the night to regroup, and the following morning the decision was made to place an additional central line in Lexi's arm. This PICC line was in addition to the Broviac line that was still in her chest. The two central lines were necessary to be able to continue with treatment and give her body the nutrition it needed through an IV. We would start again with the TPN. There was no other option.

"Hey Lexi, once you get this PICC line in, you will have had every kind of central line we do up here at Primary's," the nurse said, smiling at Lexi.

With a twinkle of life in her gaunt blue eyes, Lexi faintly smiled. "This way I will be able to relate to more people and what they are going through when I'm a nurse."

Chapter Twenty-Five

The Sufferings of This Present Time Shall Pass

(Romans 8:18)

*F*or now, the plan was to begin Lexi's fourth treatment in just a few days and to give her body IV nutrition around the clock. This was less than ideal, because Lexi's liver counts still had not returned to normal. The liver did not like TPN, and Lexi's liver was just looking for a reason to be angry. I felt like we were just poking the bear. I knew we weren't facing anything that other families of children with chronic illnesses didn't regularly face, but it felt overwhelming nonetheless. The long-term plans were still being formulated to help her digestive tract fully recover, but our energy for now had to be focused on giving her the support she needed to complete treatment.

As I pondered our current situation, my mind continued to be assaulted with the "what ifs" and "why nots." I looked at Lex and was consistently reminded of how different her life was from what I thought it would be. I thought she would be getting stronger again by now, not still fighting to survive. She should be dancing, not struggling to walk.

It was in these deepest moments of weakness, when there was nothing left, that trust entered in. Not hope or blind following, but pure trust. I trusted that Heavenly Father knew the path that her life needed to take and that He was constantly guiding her, just as

He will for each of us if we allow Him to. I trusted that her suffering, and the suffering of others, was not in vain. I trusted in the fulfillment of priesthood blessings, and I was learning to trust in the Lord's timing.

The PICC line was placed, and around-the-clock IV nutrition began. Lexi continued to eat small amounts of whatever she could eat, fighting her body with every swallow, willing it to make a comeback. Slowly her body began processing food again and her weight began to recover. Every day we saw positive ounces that eventually turned into pounds. With the weight gain came a slight increase in energy and strength. Bit by bit she improved, and the teams all agreed that she could have five days at home before returning to the hospital for her next treatment. After a month in the hospital, we were again heading to our safe haven.

It is amazing the strength that can be found in surrounding yourself with the people you love the most. During our week at home, Lexi was getting a constant infusion of medication that prepared her for round four of antibody therapy. This infusion made her feel like she had an insane case of the flu, complete with body aches, coughing, sore throat, and extreme exhaustion, but she couldn't help loving life. Her heart became rejuvenated, and she reveled in surrounding herself with those she loved so dearly.

She was home. Her days were spent on her couch, not a generic hospital bed. Cam, Liv, and Aleah could come and sit with her all at once and didn't have to leave. Family prayer was said together, in the same room every night. Hugs were given every day. Everything that went in and out of her body did not have to be measured, and she did not have to be weighed twice a day. There were no leads on her chest, no cuff on her arm, no monitor on her finger, no alarms when she slept. She was home.

Kris and I had gone on a date to celebrate our eighteenth anniversary. He had made all of the arrangements, and I was deeply thankful to be able to enjoy our time, knowing that all of our kids were at home together. Kris had always gone above and beyond when it came to our anniversary, and this year was no different. He surprised

me with matching shirts that read, "Eighteen years and still in love."
A reservation had been made at a restaurant that was completely out
of our budget, and he spoke with the woman playing the piano to
request that she play the first song we danced to as husband and wife
(which was also the same song that was playing when he kissed me
for the first time). Afterward we attended a play at our community
theatre.

The night was surreal. We laughed and joked and felt completely
carefree. Everything was right in the world once again. During inter-
mission, I called home to check on the kids and let them know what
time we would be home. "Hey, honey, how are things going?" I asked
Lexi.

"Everyone's fine. We are just having a sibling sleepover in the
front room and watching a movie."

"How fun!" I said. "Dad and I should be home in about forty-
five minutes. Love you, sweetheart."

I went to hang up, and she said, "Uh, mom?"

"Yeah?" I replied.

"I didn't want to tell you this because I didn't want to ruin
your night, but I have a fever . . . It's 102.3. I'm really sorry, Mom.
I wanted you and Dad to have a fun night and enjoy your time
together. I'm sorry I got a fever."

"Honey, we have talked about this. You only need to apologize in
life for the things you can control. You getting a fever is completely
out of your control." I went on to ask more specific questions that I
knew the doctors would need answers to when we called to tell them
about the fever. Kris and I headed home, and I called the doctor.
The symptoms she was having lined up with the side effects of her
infusion, so they allowed us to monitor her at home for the night.
How grateful I was that we were able to once again kneel together for
prayer in the same room that evening.

Lexi's fevers persisted on throughout the night, the following
day spiking to 103.1 degrees Fahrenheit. Her symptoms continued
to escalate, and the doctors decided it was time to bring her in. We
headed to the hospital yet again, where antibiotics were administered

and tests were performed. She had caught the flu. Luckily, she had an inkling of an immune system, so we were allowed to go home with additional medication and instruction.

"Her fever got high enough that I'm not sure that the team will feel comfortable going on with treatment," the on-call doctor told us. "Antibody is a treatment that puts the immune system on ultimate high alert. It is over-stimulated, so it attacks everything and anything. With her body having this virus, it would amplify all of the effects of the antibody therapy. This means that if we go through with the treatment, she will experience heightened side effects from an already difficult treatment. Honestly, with what her body has already been through, I'm not sure if it could handle that with the current state she's in. Even if there were a way that she could, I'm not sure she'd even want to. It would be that bad."

I wanted to be done with treatment, but not at the risk of my child suffering more than she needed to. However, Lexi lobbied to move forward.

Again the doctor reiterated the increased effects, to which Lexi countered, "I want to do it. I've done hard things before. I can do anything for five days." We were discharged with the knowledge that the team would make a final decision and get back to us in a few hours as to how we would proceed.

Lexi's wish was granted, and that Monday we traveled to the hospital for round four of antibody therapy. During our drive up to the hospital, the song "Unanswered Prayers" came on the radio. I sang along without realizing it as my mind was focused on what this week would hold, praying that she could withstand the storm that promised to rage. After the song was over, Lex said, "Mom, I don't believe that any prayer goes unanswered. I think that sometimes the answer is yes, sometimes it is no, and sometimes the timing just isn't right. God does not just 'not answer' when we talk to Him. Just because we may not get the answer that we want does not mean that our prayers are unanswered."

Over the course of this treatment, I had seen tangible evidence of God in our lives, yet there had still been times that it felt as if He may not have heard every prayer I uttered. We had traveled down paths I would rather have avoided and prayed to be spared from situations that we never wanted to be in. However, during our darkest hour, when there were a million reasons to doubt, we kept searching for the one reason to believe, because it was always there. He was always there, and that knowledge was what kept us going strong.

We parked the car and headed to a familiar room on the fourth floor. It was no longer the dreaded ICS unit or "the cancer floor." It was our second home. It was a place where we were welcomed with bright smiles and warm embraces, where Lexi was asked about dates and dances and the cute boys at school. It was a place where I was asked about how Kris, Cam, Liv, and Aleah were doing—by name. It was a place where I could talk openly about the horrors I was afraid to show the rest of the world for fear that they were actually real. It was a place that understood me when I rambled and saw beauty in me when I hadn't slept in days. It was a place that loved me when I was broken and held me while my child healed. It is true that there is no place like home, but if there were, it would be this place.

We quickly settled into our familiar surroundings, and the antibody medication took no time proving that it would be more of a challenge than Lexi had previously conquered. High fevers, high blood pressure, low blood pressure, hives, respiratory issues, elevated heart rate, blood transfusions, and, of course, extreme pain all combined to launch an attack on her fragile body. It seemed the time could not pass quickly enough for her next dose of Tylenol to be administered. It wouldn't completely break the fevers, but once every few hours it would line up with a few other meds, and when combined with cold washcloths on her head, it proved to offer some relief.

However, when people asked her how she was doing, Lexi's response was always the same. "I'm healthy enough to start treatment again, so I am good." She truly was so grateful to be moving forward and nearing the end of her treatment. Lexi did not focus on her setbacks, only that she was able to keep progressing toward her goal.

Written on the whiteboard in her room was one of her favorite scriptures. "For I reckon that the sufferings of this present time are not worthy to be compared to the glory that shall be revealed in us" (Romans 8:18). The words rang especially true for her at this time, and she held closely to the promise of great things to come.

Like all difficult trials, our week came to an end. We left the hospital with a new appreciation for the word "exhausted." But the excitement of being home combined with the knowledge that we had only one more hospital stay fueled our hearts. We were almost done . . . or so we thought.

Lexi had a great weekend and was able to spend some time with friends, attend all of church for the first time in months, and even watch the Super Bowl with some of her favorite people. She was doing better and looking better, and we were so very thankful to finally have a straight shot to the finish line. However, cancer had taught us nothing if not that things could change instantaneously.

Early Tuesday morning, after being home for just over three days, Lex began vomiting large quantities of bright red blood. I took a picture of the contents of our toilet and called the hospital while grabbing an overnight bag. She needed to be admitted right away, so we woke our kids to tell them that Lexi and I needed to leave. We had family prayer and said our good-byes, with no indication of how soon we would be back home.

The doctors assessed Lexi, looked at the picture on my phone, and came to the conclusion that she was experiencing internal bleeding. She was given multiple platelet and blood transfusions. This combined with prayers and pleadings on her behalf allowed the bleeding to desist. However, she began struggling with unexplained high blood pressure, headaches, and increased amounts of pain. Many different tests and imaging were completed in order to rule things out. New medications were added, and some meds were stopped.

"You know, Lexi," one of the doctors said in jest, "you just like to challenge us and keep us on our toes. Over the past five weeks, you have had pneumonia, influenza, and an antibody treatment; your GI tract has shut down; you've had RSV; and all this is in addition to whatever is going on right now."

She looked back to them with a sheepish grin. "It's because I am such a high-maintenance girl."

The doctors had come to know her too well to believe that. "No, we just need to work harder to find the problem. We should have it worked out so you can be home in just a few days."

Lexi smiled patiently at them, fully understanding that cancer operates in its own time zone. She then responded with, "I don't love the hospital, but I can stay as long as I am home within twelve days." She answered their quizzical looks by finishing with, "I have a sweethearts dance that I really need to get to." They smiled and remembered that while she was a cancer patient, she was also still a teenage girl. They agreed to do their best to see that discharge happened before then.

The monotony of hospital life was broken by a special visit from Sister Jones, the general Primary president, and Sister Peay, the Relief Society president of the PCMC branch. Sister Peay and her husband made regular visits to whichever room we found ourselves in and often brought inspired messages with them. They had become more than a spiritual strength on this journey. They were dear friends that we looked forward to seeing. Their visits always lightened our load and filled our hearts.

On this day, Lexi had the opportunity to visit directly with Sister Jones, and it was a phenomenal experience. We visited and spoke of things that were happening and the direction we were hoping to be headed in. The spirit in the room was tangible, and our burdens felt lighter as we enjoyed one another's company. Embraces were given, and the two sisters left. Lexi was beaming as the door closed behind them.

"That was pretty amazing, sis," I told her.

"I know . . . ," she said, halfway lost in her own thoughts. "You know when you and Sister Peay were visiting and I was talking with Sister Jones?"

"Yes," I said.

"She told me things that were promised to me in blessings and talked about this trial and what it would hold for my life." She paused. "She said things word for word that had been spoken in blessings and even in my patriarchal blessing."

Lexi went on to tell me that Sister Jones said that Lexi's experiences and testimony had already changed more lives than she realized. She said she would continue to change many lives. Sister Jones had told Lexi, "You have some very specific and important things you will do on this earth one day." She had then paused and looked intently at Lex. "But you already know and understand that, don't you?" Lex had just smiled softly and nodded, humbled by this special exchange and grateful for the unique interaction and testimony that came with it. Many times it is hard to see the impact we have on the lives of others when our days are spent in solitude.

We had been gone from home for a week now. Each night held the promise of the possibility of going home, and each morning that possibility eluded us. Many times before, I had felt the effect that cancer had on a family as a whole. There had been times when Lexi had mentioned that certain things were harder on her siblings than they were on her. One such time came for our youngest, Aleah, as she asked yet again when we would be home. She'd had enough of her sister and me being gone. She was a very analytical young woman who loved learning and knowing things, the kind of girl who works best with consistency and a firm schedule. Cancer offered no such things.

Aleah had been struggling with the uncertainty of when we would and would not be home. The last few months had been spent as much at home as in the hospital. Her frustration was apparent in her nightly text, which read, "Mommy I wish that you could always be at home and tuck me in because I miss it so much. I love you and HATE that you have to be gone. I hate it so much that I would rather give up my room than have anyone in our family have cancer." These were pretty powerful words for a nine-year-old.

My heart longed to be there with her, to hold her while she cried and tell her that it would be okay. We were so close to being done, but Aleah's young heart had taken all it could. I tried to comfort her the best I could from a distance, but it was not what she needed. She needed to be held and know that everything would be okay, but I couldn't be there to do it. My fragile mom heart broke into miniscule pieces. I knew what she needed, and I knew I couldn't fulfill that need. There are few things in life that will render a greater pain in the heart of a parent than being told by her child that she is hurting and not being able to do anything to help ease that suffering. A feeling of utter helplessness washed over me. I quietly wept with despair as I sent the most uplifting text I could muster and waited for her response.

About fifteen minutes passed, and I got another text. "Me and Dad just got done cuddling, and I'm going to go to bed, so I love you, good night."

Kris continued to be a rock for our family, fighting to keep any sense of normalcy that could exist amidst this chaos. But he did so much more than meet the temporal needs of our children. He picked up the pieces of our broken hearts and held them while they healed. As I was thanking my Father in Heaven for the amazing blessing Kris was in our lives, I learned an eternal lesson. I realized that there would be times in my children's lives that they would be sad. They would experience heartache, and as much as I wanted to be there and hold them, I wouldn't always be able to.

There would be times when I knew what they needed but would not be able to help, and times that I would have to watch helplessly, unaware of what their needs might be. Gratitude filled my soul as I realized that even when I could not be there to hold them, they had an Eternal Father who knew and fully understood every scenario they would face and every feeling that would accompany their life. A loving Heavenly Father would forever be there to comfort and strengthen them. I knew this to be true, because I had felt it myself.

I had felt the loneliness and the sorrow, the despair and desperation. I had cried out that I hated our circumstances and would give anything to not have to face them anymore. I had begged for my family to just be together again. But ultimately I found myself cradled in the arms of my Father as He lovingly held me until I felt strong enough to stand back up and carry on.

Prayers were answered, and I made it home to hold my baby girl. Lexi made it home in time to attend her sweethearts dance. She spent the day with her friends and danced into the night. We were home for almost four days before heading back to the hospital for her last inpatient stay. After this stay, Lexi would have to continue with her oral chemo and then officially start the uphill battle of recovery. It would be a long, difficult road, but it was one that we were very grateful to travel.

Chapter Twenty-Six

I Can Do All Things through Christ
(Philippians 4:13)

*F*our good night kisses and four good morning hugs were not enough, but we took solace knowing that our days apart were numbered. This was it—Lexi's official last inpatient hospital stay. Soon there would be no more calls from clinic saying we would unexpectedly be staying inpatient, no more keeping an overnight bag in the car, no more counting how many days until we had to be apart again, and no more watching grasped hands slowly tear apart through rolled-down windows as we drove away amidst tear-streaked faces.

Over the course of seventeen months, we had spent more than 330 days in the hospital. For many of those days, Lexi had been confined to a small room, unable to leave, and was limited in who she could have contact with. Multiple chemo medications had coursed through her small veins. She had undergone four major surgeries—three on an emergency basis. Her bone marrow had been wiped clean with fatal chemotherapy and then restored—twice. She had endured radiation and battled through antibody therapy. She had received more than 130 life-saving transfusions. Her body had sustained more damage, and her heart had taken more hits than most would ever need to comprehend, but we were finally here.

Tears filled my eyes, and thankfulness filled my heart as I looked at my daughter. She had oxygen to help her breathe and seven pumps delivering her last infusion. I took her hand and touched her precious newly grown hair. "I'm so proud of you, honey. You did it," I softly whispered.

With love in her eyes, she looked at me and said, "No, Mama, *we* did it. We all did it—together." I held her as the last of the infusion, the last treatment, the last hit to her armor was delivered.

The next day we were discharged, with plans to only come back to clinic. No more hospital stays, no more medications. We had not been home for longer than ten consecutive days in the last four months. We would finally break our record. We would sleep in our own beds and give good morning kisses and good night loves. We were on the road to the rest of our lives.

Lexi began to slowly improve and was doing well enough that she was able to visit clinic once every two weeks. "I am now in the 'take back my life' part of my fight song!" She proclaimed with great enthusiasm. She returned to school full time for the fourth quarter of her junior year.

"How is school life going, babe?" I asked after school one day.

"I feel lucky to go, Mama, but it's hard."

"Don't stress about it," I said. "You're smart and motivated. I know you can catch up in time to walk with your class at graduation."

"It's not just that," she replied. "I'm really excited to be at school, but I'm also really nervous and a little scared. Everyone has changed and I haven't been there. My friends have inside jokes that I'm not a part of, and I don't know where or if I fit in. I feel like I'm ready to start doing normal things again, but my hair is still really short and I'm still really skinny. I feel like I still look like the sick kid, and I don't want to be treated any differently." She paused and then added, "But I know I'm not the same that I was."

Slowly she began her return to dancing, doing as much as her body would allow. Her weight proved to be a struggle that she would battle. Months later, we would learn that this was a consequence of her pancreas ceasing to function as a result of treatment and her body not being able to apply the nutrition from the food that she ate. To combat this, she would need to take enzymes each time she ate for the rest of her life.

During a routine clinic visit, Lexi's doctor talked about how far she had come and how far she still had to go. "I'm so proud of you, Lex! You are on your way to going back to normal life." She paused slightly before continuing on. "You are making great progress and are on your way back to having a normal life. Just remember that cancer changes things, Lex. It'll never be like it was before."

That hit me hard. For the past year and a half, we had lived in survival mode, and I'd longed for the time that we could return to normal life. I now understood that there was no such thing as "normal life." Just life. If I spent my time longing for days past, hoping they would replay in future days, then this experience would have been in vain. There would always be trials and difficult times, but that was where so much growth took place. It was amid our greatest challenges that our true character was revealed.

My hopes for no more hospital stays were in vain. We had made it just over three weeks at home when Lexi began running an insanely high fever. Although treatment had been completed and Lexi's PICC line had been removed, she still had her Broviac line in order to deliver her TPN. Running a fever with a central line in place is extremely dangerous, because it can allow an infection to travel quite quickly throughout the entirety of the bloodstream. We headed back to clinic, unsure of the cause of this sudden fever.

A viral panel was run to check and see the source of the fever. It came back negative, so it was assumed that what she had contracted was bacterial. She was given a dose of Tylenol to help break the fever, and forty-five minutes later it spiked to 104.7 degrees Fahrenheit. "Hey," she said, slightly delusional from the fever, "that's a new high score for me!" The medical team did not share her enthusiasm.

Lexi began having severe chills and body aches. She began to shake as I tried to soothe her. Her blood pressure dropped to 80/42. Her labs had just come back and showed that her kidney numbers had increased by 50 percent in the last three days and that her liver numbers were elevated as well. She continued to become progressively weaker in what felt like a matter of minutes. "What can cause this sudden onset of such extreme symptoms?" I asked the doctor, not even trying to mask the fear in my voice.

She looked at Lexi's shaking frame and replied, "It is probable that the bacteria is trying to enter her blood stream and take over. Her body is likely going septic."

I went numb. I had heard that term, and it was never associated with a positive outcome. Multiple antibiotics were given to Lexi intravenously, and two nurses were asked to look after her. I had logged enough hours on the cancer floor to know that the general ratio of nurses to patients is typically one nurse to every two patients, sometimes three. The more experienced nurses are given the transplant and antibody kiddos. This is usually done on a one-to-one ratio. Two nurses had just been asked to look after Lexi. Throughout all of treatment, that had never happened. I didn't want to think what that meant.

We settled in our room as the doctor kept looking from Lexi to the monitor and back to Lexi. The more experienced nurse told the doctor to relax, but she just kept staring at Lexi with a furrowed brow, trying to figure out what to do next. "The problem is that we are running out of options with Lexi. If she goes down, she is going down quick."

I again was grateful for the knowledge that we have been given that Lexi would never go down farther than she could climb back up. I also decided that while I appreciated honesty, I also appreciated delicate wording. Apparently, you can't have both. Everyone left our room with the same phrase: "Let's just hope that tonight is uneventful."

"Do you ever sleep up here?" the nurse asked when she came to get Lexi's vitals just fifteen minutes after she had taken them before.

"Does anyone really sleep up here?" I answered with a wry smile. "How is she doing?" I asked, although I already knew. I had learned how to take vitals, read monitors, and understand saturation levels months before. If not, I would have worried myself into a coma.

"She's progressively getting a little bit better every time we come in, but something tells me you would have had us come check sooner if she weren't," she said with an understanding smile. "Try to get some rest, Em. She'll be okay, and she'll be worried if she knows you were up all night again." I smiled, not only at the concern my sweet friend had for me, but also for how well she knew the relationship and the love that Lex and I had for each other. She was right, of course. Lex would ask how I slept in the morning, and it was no secret that I was a terrible liar. I closed my eyes and did my best to get some hospital rest.

Our prayers were answered, and the night proved to be very uneventful. Lexi continued to have severe body aches but began to describe them as recovery pain. I still did not love that she had experienced so much pain that she knew how to distinguish one from the other. She had not run a fever for almost twelve hours and seemed to be responding well to the continued medication. Her heart rate had returned to normal, and her counts were slowly heading in the right direction. If she was able to continue on this path, there was talk of sending us home as early as the following day. Again she was a mystery. The doctors were still not sure what brought on her symptoms, but we knew why they were clearing up. Again, our lives had been blessed by the power of prayer.

I would be lying if I said that I did not plead with my Heavenly Father that we might be spared this hospital stay. My heart yearned to stay at home longer, to enjoy the weekend we had planned as a family. As I was taking my mandated walk to the cafeteria, I passed by this amazing tree with flowers so beautiful I had to touch them to believe they were actually real.

A man saw me admiring the tree and said, "That is a magnolia tree. It doesn't always bloom like that. If we get a late frost or it's not warm early enough in the spring, it won't turn out to be as beautiful as this. The timing and conditions all have to be right for it to reach its full potential." I thanked the man for sharing his knowledge, sure that he had no idea how much it was needed at the time.

I smiled and realized that if God took the time to help that beautiful tree reach its full potential, then I could trust that He would do nothing less for us. I did not always understand the conditions we were asked to live, but I had finally come to fully trust in the timing of the Lord and was in awe at the masterpiece He could make of each of our lives. We just needed to understand and have the patience that He was making sure that the conditions were perfect for us to flourish. I picked a fragrant blossom and brought it back to Lexi. As she was admiring the beauty of the flower, I thanked my Heavenly Father for taking the time to make sure that our conditions were perfect for us to blossom when I had been praying for the exact opposite.

Lexi continued to improve, and we were sent home. She had one more week of oral chemo left, and then her end of treatment scans would follow just a few weeks later. Oral chemo was much less intrusive on the body, but still held its own difficulties. The oral chemo that she was on was known as Accutane. Many people take this to treat acne. Essentially what it did was slow the blood supply to fast-growing cells, causing them to dry out. Research had proven that when given in high doses it could also limit the blood supply to cancer cells (as they were fast growing as well), thus causing them to die.

The normal dosage for Accutane was one pill a day. Lexi had been taking six pills a day for two weeks each month for the past six months. When she began this regimen, the doctors told us that they could give us the normal side effects of this particular treatment for a child five or under, but they had no idea how Lexi would react, because they had never placed a teen on this treatment. Normal side effects included extremely dry skin, mood swings, and depression. We felt grateful that Lexi only experienced the dry skin and depression, but her depression was such that it more than made up for the lack of mood swings.

The doctors had told us that a cancer patient was three times more likely to experience depression. It was also well known that cancer survivors could suffer from post-traumatic stress disorder (PTSD) and survivor's guilt. It seemed to be that they all combined to launch a full-blown attack on Lexi's psyche simultaneously. She struggled to overcome the assault and decided to put measures in place for the extremely tough times. Lexi held close to her patriarchal blessing, limited her time on social media, attended the temple often, prayed, and held on with all her might as her trial switched from a physical fight to a mental battle. This stage proved to have many challenges, but like the rest of this journey, they were met head on and slowly overcome.

We had been home together, with the exception of clinic visits, for a few weeks, and we were ABSOLUTELY LOVING IT! We had lived apart for so long that we were readjusting to life together all the time now. Not a day passed that we didn't thank Heavenly Father that this was something we were blessed to experience. It was springtime now, and I had the opportunity to take my girls to listen to the semiannual women's session of general conference. Many of the talks given spoke of trials that others were facing. Cancer, in particular, seemed to play a central role. I have to admit that I felt a little vulnerable when some emotions expressed were still so raw in my fragile heart. However, something greater than heaviness of heart entered my soul.

Lexi had been asked multiple times that if she could choose, would she make the decision to not have cancer? Her response was always the same: "Cancer was the hardest thing I've ever had to face. It's harder than anyone knows or could even understand, but I've learned things I know I couldn't have learned any other way. I wouldn't change a thing. I know that God is real. I know that miracles are real. These aren't beliefs but real knowledge. God gives us trials to make us stronger. He does it because He loves us. Without our trials, we wouldn't be who God needs us to be. We should never take anything for granted but be grateful for every moment of our lives. We have to trust God. He has a plan. I know He does, even when it feels like He doesn't. We can look for the good in every situation and look for God in every situation. He is always there, even if we have to look a little harder sometimes."

I can't say that if given the choice I would choose to watch my child suffer in hopes of gaining a deeper understanding of eternal truths. My imperfect heart could sacrifice myself, but not my child. I can, however, appreciate that whether it is cancer or any other trial, lessons can be learned during our difficult times that cannot be learned any other way. We can spend our time being frustrated or angry about where we are. We can cry and scream that our situation is unfair, and many times it is. We can quietly weep as we feel our hearts literally breaking at the load we are asked to bear. Trust me, I've been there. Or we can choose to allow ourselves to be taught the lessons that are unique to the situations we are in. The most amazing part is that the choice is ours. We are not being forced into learning or acceptance of our situation. We are given a choice.

I am not saying one approach is preferable to the other. Each trial and situation is unique to the person or family going through it. Sometimes crying is what's needed; other times remaining positive is key. The trick is to understand that while we might be facing so many obstacles that are completely out of our control, there will always be one thing that we can control: our response to the situation. Ultimately our happiness is in our hands, and those hands can always clasp together in prayer.

Not a day passes that I don't look at each of my children and thank God for the miracle that they are, for the miracle of hearing their laughter in the morning or seeing their freckles in the sun. However, there are still days when a dark cloud threatens to hang overhead, blocking my sunlight. We have seen so much sadness and gloom and so many families torn apart so many times by this disease that we have no guarantee that it will not happen again to our own.

When these thoughts threaten to launch their assault on my happiness, I am reminded that the uncertainty of the future is not limited to cancer patients and their families. Mortality is something that we each face every day. We do not know the last time we will kiss our loved ones good-bye, or the last time we will all be together as families. Nothing is guaranteed. In the cancer world, this reality is brought to the forefront, forcing us to make the most of each beautiful day. But shouldn't we be taking this opportunity every day? Life is delicate and difficult. It is beautiful and chaotic, but it is our life to live. We cannot choose how long we live, only *how* we live. If I have learned anything, it is that life is a gift, an amazingly fragile gift. Live it. Love it. Never, ever take it for granted. Perhaps this is one of the most important things I have learned: life is full of beauty when we choose to look for the wildflowers instead of focusing on the weeds.

The sky began to release the rain it had been holding hostage, bringing me back to the present day. The dark clouds still loomed overhead as the storm threatened to worsen, and yet it just made me search for the sun with a renewed energy. It was there, I knew it was, I knew it would be. I knew it always had been. A warmth washed over me as an overwhelming peace painted itself into every memory, every tear shed, every prayer offered, and every heartache felt. An understanding came. Perhaps we were given this storm to more clearly see the Son, to seek Him out, appreciate Him more fully, and understand the need for Him in our everyday lives. Our storm clouds didn't keep us from the warmth of the Son but gave us the understanding that even in our darkest times there is light to be found.

Epilogue

Scans had been completed, and we were waiting to hear the final results. Even though all of Lexi's imaging since surgery had been clear, the anxiety brought on by scans (known by cancer parents as "scanxiety") was surreal. Kris had come to clinic with us to hear what we hoped would be the end of this journey. The doctor entered the room, and the tightening in my chest reminded me that oxygen was still important. I let out the breath I had been subconsciously holding.

The doctor grabbed a stool and sat down. "Let's skip to the end, and then we can go over each individual test . . . All of her scans are clear. There is no evidence of disease in Lexi's body."

My lip quivered, and Kris's shoulders seemed to visibly lighten. I looked over to see Lexi's clear blue eyes shining. The truths she'd known in her heart were finally aligning with what she was being told. The doctor then passed on the results of the tests to us. "Lexi's bone marrow is at 60 percent right now. We would like to see it around 80 percent, but we have put her through the ringer and then some, so we feel like 60 percent is acceptable for now. Her platelets are still struggling to recover, and we are not sure why. We are hoping that over time they will continue to get stronger. Her lung function is a little worse than it was the last time we checked. This isn't surprising, because her lungs have struggled for over a year now, and the treatment is known to damage them further. We will be referring her to a pulmonologist for further monitoring."

He paused to ask us if we had any questions. We shook our heads, and he continued on. "Her heart is functioning on the very low end of normal, so she will have repeat echocardiograms to monitor her condition. Her heart and lungs may improve, but only time will tell." He continued with the many side effects that would be permanent—just the price she would pay to live.

The results and effects had all been covered, and our few questions had been answered. The doctor looked over to Lexi caringly. "You know, the fact that we get to have this conversation with these results is really something amazing. Given where you were, and what you've been through, I wasn't sure we would get here. We could have been having a much different conversation today." My heart swelled with gratitude that it was not the conversation we were having today. A sharp pain quickly followed for the parents who *had* had that conversation.

Regardless of the damage done to her body and the uphill climb of recovery, Lexi remained grateful for the health she had and the opportunity to be able to continue living her life. She was able to ring the bell, just as Jake did, declaring that she was done with treatment and cancer free.

Lexi enrolled in school full time and was able to serve as an officer on her drill team for her senior year. As she continued to improve, we began to make our transition from the cancer world back to the typical world. There were days when this came easy, and days that the emotion of this journey still felt suffocating. My heart remains humbled for the rare opportunity we had to grow and learn together as a family and for the patience of a loving Heavenly Father who allowed us to do so.

Today, Lexi is one year cancer free. Her doctors refer to her as an "anomaly for many reasons, but especially in the cancer world." She worked hard to make up the credits she missed from being sick so that she could graduate with her class, and she will begin college in the fall. She is majoring in nursing and plans on working in a pediatric oncology unit.

Lexi says that while cancer took many things from her, it gave her something even better in return—her best friend, Ricky—the tall boy with the dark hair and the warm smile who danced to make

Lexi laugh in the cancer clinic. Over the course of her treatment, he would continue to find ways to bring joy into her life, and she would bring strength into his. He visited her regularly at the hospital to play games, sing to her, or just hang out. Over time they realized that their love for one another extended far beyond friendship. On September 15, 2018, they were married in the Mount Timpanogos Utah Temple. Their story is one for the ages, but that is a tale for another time.

Acknowledgments

With deepest gratitude, we wish to thank the doctors, surgeons, nurses, techs, imaging department, cleaning and cafeteria employees, and each member of the staff at Primary Children's Hospital. Each of you played a vital role in Lexi's journey and the healing of our family.

Our deepest love and appreciation to the LDS branch at Primary Children's Hospital for the genuine love and concern with which you fulfill your calling. Thank you for caring for our hearts and spirits at such a tender time.

Much love to our Magna community. You are family. You have supported and loved our children as your own. You have carried Kris and me when we were too weak to stand. Thank you for showing us time and again that we were truly never alone in this fight. Once a pirate, always a pirate.

To each member of our family: Words cannot express our gratitude for your kindness, patience, and understanding with us as we traveled through uncharted territory. Thank you for loving and trusting us enough to know that we would make it, even when we doubted it ourselves. There aren't words to express what your love means to us, especially during this time. We love each of you and humbly thank Heavenly Father that He allows us to be a part of your lives.

We humbly wish to acknowledge all those who have ever been affected by this disease in any capacity, as well as their loved ones. Thank you, my friends, for teaching us how to love, how to laugh, how to cry, how to rebuild, and how to endure. Cancer brought some of our dearest friends into our lives, and although it took some of them back, we will always carry them in our hearts.

About the Author

Emily Gould

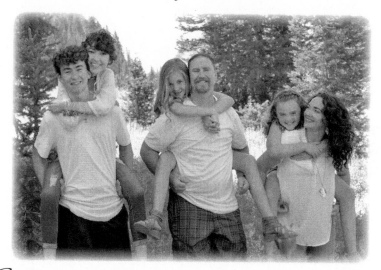

*E*mily Gould has been writing for over twenty years. Within the last few years, she has enjoyed writing various columns and covering local events for the *Magna Times*. She is currently the editor and publisher of this local newspaper. Upon her daughter's cancer diagnosis, writing became less of a hobby and more of a coping mechanism that Emily used to understand and learn more about herself and the unfamiliar situations her family found themselves in.

With her husband, Kris, by her side, Emily is always up for any adventure that life has to offer. The couple, along with their four children, enjoy camping, hiking, boating, laughing too loud, and just being together.

About the Author

Alexis Gould Stafford

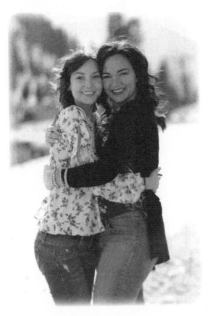

lexis Gould Stafford was a healthy teenage girl until her world changed without warning. She went to the ER thinking her appendix had burst, only to learn that she had a life-threatening form of cancer and her tumor had ruptured. Her unwillingness to give up despite unfavorable odds, coupled with her humor in dire circumstances, caused her story to spread quickly, and she became known as #AlexisStrong.

Alexis is passionate about spreading awareness of childhood cancer and the truths she has learned through cancer. She enjoys sharing her story, the miracles she has witnessed, the heartache she has felt, the hope she holds, and the very real love of God she knows exists as often as she can.

Scan to visit

www.emilygouldwrites.com